The Ethics of Gender-Specific Disease

Routledge Annals of Bioethics

Series Editors: MARK J. CHERRY, *St. Edward's University, USA*
ANA SMITH ILTIS, *Wake Forest University, USA*

The Ethics of
Gender-Specific Disease

Mary Ann G. Cutter

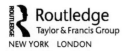

Routledge
Taylor & Francis Group
NEW YORK   LONDON

First published 2012
by Routledge
711 Third Avenue, New York, NY 10017

Simultaneously published in the UK
by Routledge
2 Park Square, Milton Park, Abingdon, Oxon OX14 4RN

*Routledge is an imprint of the Taylor & Francis Group,
an informa business*

Library of Congress Cataloging-in-Publication Data
Cutter, Mary Ann Gardell.
   The ethics of gender-specific disease / Mary Ann G. Cutter.
      p. cm. — (Routledge annals of bioethics)
   Includes bibliographical references (p. 131) and index.
   1.   Medical ethics.   2.   Sex factors in disease.   3.   Health—Sex
differences.   I. Title.
   R725.5.C88 2012
   174.2'969—dc23
   2011040736

ISBN: 978-0-415-50997-8 (hbk)
ISBN: 978-0-203-12342-3 (ebk)

Typeset in Sabon
by IBT Global.

To my father, John Patrick Gardell, who knew well before the popularity of second-wave feminism that women deserved better. His support and encouragement have made projects like this possible.

Contents

Preface

We begin with some words of advice:

> Sometimes diseases become incurable for women who do not learn why they are sick before the doctor has been correctly taught by the sick women why she is sick. For women are shamed to tell even of their inexperience and lack of knowledge. At the same time the doctors also make mistakes by not learning the apparent cause through accurate questioning, but they proceed to heal as though they were dealing with men's diseases. I have already seen many women die from just this kind of suffering. But at the outset one must ask accurate questions about the cause. For the healing of the diseases of women differs greatly from the healing of men's diseases (Hippocrates 2005 [fifth c. B.C.E.], 62).

The insight that gender matters in disease expression and treatment is not new. Long ago in the fifth century, the notable Ancient Greek physician Hippocrates shared his observation that "the healing of the diseases of women differs greatly from the healing of men's diseases" (Hippocrates 2005, 62). Despite Hippocrates' observation in the clinic, western medicine has historically given little attention to gender-specific differences in disease expression and treatment. With the recent rise of gender-specific medicine, and its sub-specialty women's health care, things have begun to change.

Today, medical professionals and patients are increasingly aware that there are important gender differences in the symptoms, frequencies, diagnosis, prognosis, and treatment of disease. Obviously, there are important gender differences in reproductive problems. Ovarian cancer is found only in women and testicular cancer only in men. Breast cancer affects far more women than men, even though men are known to express breast cancer. In addition to the reproductive problems, there is much to explore. There is little disagreement that, among women and men, some diseases have different symptoms (e.g., in the case of AIDS), different frequencies (e.g., in the case of lupus), different diagnoses (e.g., in the case of cardiovascular disease), different prognoses (e.g., in the case of lung disease), and different treatments (e.g., in the case of hypothyroidism).

Although gender differences in disease expression and treatment have become notable, there are significant ethical challenges in this new field of medicine. Part of the challenge in gendering disease has to do with defining the concept itself. Is gender-specific disease discovered or created? Is it simply a function of disclosing the difference that chromosomes make in disease expression or is it a trendy classification created in order to address past failures to study diseases that affect women in unique ways and to advocate for alternative ways? Is gender-specific disease value-neutral or value-ladened? Is it simply a "fact" disclosed by clinical scientists or is it an "evaluation" of biomedical dysfunction by clinicians and patients? Is gender-specific disease local or global in its reach? Is it a clinical category that makes sense only in particular contexts or one that transcends local knowledge communities that can be used in the service of global medicine? Whereas these questions paint a simplistic picture of the options, we are left with important questions: What is gender-specific disease? How do we know it? What role, if any, do values play in the clinical category? These and related questions are explored in this inquiry.

Why, one might ask, should anyone care about a philosophical analysis of gender-specific disease? The short answer is that confusion about the nature of gender-specific disease is confusion about gender-specific medicine itself. An errant account of gender-specific disease can lead to overgeneralizations, undergeneralizations, and/or mislabels of clinical conditions that affect members of certain genders. This can lead to inaccurate diagnostic and treatment recommendations for patients, which can affect how we write health policies and health laws and develop clinical curricula and health care delivery systems. How we understand gender-specific disease turns on a whole set of assumptions and claims about the nature of clinical reality, how we know it, and how we value it. It further affects how medicine is practiced and patient lives are changed. Put another way, there are significant ethical implications of how gender-specific disease is understood. This important aspect of the discussion is also explored in this inquiry.

The impetus for this project on the ethics of gender-specific disease is a consequence of numerous forces. First, I spent a fair amount of my early scholarly work in philosophy on the historical and conceptual development of the clinical classification of AIDS as a case study of how medicine understands disease. In the late 1980s, I, along with many others, watched the infection rates in Houston, Texas, rise and questioned how medicine ought to respond to this new clinical phenomenon. Medical history unfolded and we had front seat, so to speak. I began writing on how medical "facts" developed and transformed how we know and intervene in medicine. In 1993, I was shocked by the revelation that the U.S. Centers for Disease Control had only begun to collect data on women with AIDS. How could medicine have assumed that women were *not* infected by HIV? What were some of the claims about women that went into such calculations? How have women and their children been affected by this oversight (or rather undersight)? I began to wonder what gender-specific medicine might learn from previous errors of miscalculating the role gender plays in disease expression and treatment.

Second, my training in the philosophy of medicine, bioethics, and applied ethics in the late 1970s and early 1980s at the Kennedy Institute of Ethics at Georgetown University occurred largely without any consideration of how medicine addresses gender issues. Yet, I have "grown up" in medicine, so to speak, as a woman, writing about medicine, bearing children, taking family members to doctors, and growing older, and I have pondered similarities and differences between what I have read in the philosophy of medicine, bioethical, applied ethical, and clinical literatures that formed the basis of my training and what I have experienced first hand in the clinic and hospital as a patient, daughter, wife, mother, and friend. My reflections on this sort of training influence this work and have led me to explore further the concept of gender-specific disease. What follows is an attempt to bring together some of the traditional philosophy of medicine literature on disease with more recent discussions of gender in medicine found in feminist ontological, epistemological, bioethical, and sociological literature in order to forge a needed dialogue about the character of gender-specific disease.

Third, the rise of the new field called gender-specific medicine provides an opportunity to bring together my reflections over these past few decades. My long-time interest in clinical nosology or taxonomy (i.e., clinical classification), clinical nosography (i.e., clinical description), and clinical nomenclature (i.e., clinical language) reawakened when I began to read literature about gender-specific disease. I was struck with how some researchers and clinicians would write about gender-specific disease as a concept that can simply be discovered through a value-neutral, acontextual biomedical model. (A similar situation occurs in the genetic medical literature.) I realized that such a "reductionist" view is a product of influential forces in modern and contemporary medicine concerning the nature of knowledge, but it still gave me pause. I reflected upon how much of the hard work of philosophers of medicine on disease and gender has largely been ignored in clinical discussions of gender-specific disease. This led me again to wonder about why and how medicine missed the boat, so to speak, on properly understanding AIDS and menopause in the late twentieth century. What's the possibility that gender-specific medicine would repeat a pattern of stereotyping women and their diseases using remnants of views that are no longer sustainable? How can we ensure that gender-specific medicine promotes and protects the health of women from womb to tomb?

Fourth, the past three decades have witnessed an explosion of interest in bioethics in part because of pressing questions raised about the use of new knowledge and technology in medicine. Here bioethics, as the study of the ethical or moral implications of biomedical advances and practices, has served medicine well, for medicine has been a recipient of rich and practically fruitful discussions about reproductive rights, care for those at the end of life, and access to health care, to name a few. But I worry that this explosion has directed interest toward numerous applied issues in health care at the cost of the conceptual issues that frame them. This is the case in part because of our culture's appetite for quick, practical answers to difficult questions and our culture's penchant toward addressing ethical violations without an appreciation of the context in which ethical values and principles operate. This work on gender-specific disease is offered as a contribution to thinking about methodologies in bioethical thinking in ways that draw attention to the complex conceptual claims that frame them.

The foregoing has led me to offer this philosophical analysis of the ethics of gender-specific disease. The project argues that gender-specific disease and related bioethical discourses are philosophically *integrative*. Gender-specific disease is integrative because the *descriptive* roles of gender, disease, and their relation are inextricably tied to their *prescriptive* roles. Descriptions, observations, or the "facts" of gender-specific disease are discovered in the sense that we do not completely make up clinical reality, and they are created in the sense that we bring to our descriptions frames or lenses through which we "see" our world. Further, clinical descriptions are ordered around prescriptive or evaluative judgments, including those concerning what objects are assigned significance and what actions are appropriate and warranted in order to achieve certain medical goals. Here, the goals of medicine vary, and include minimizing pain and suffering, returning a patient to biological functioning, meeting patient demands, satisfying professional interests, securing funding, developing health policies, determining financial reimbursement, maintaining cultural and social norms, and so on. In this way, gender-specific descriptions and prescriptions are located in particular contexts. There are no timeless or non-contextual accounts of gender-specific disease, or at least there are no such interpretations available to humans. Yet, this is not a plea for disease relativism. An integrative approach sees gender-specific disease as biological dysfunction brought about by gender-specific factors explained via etiological laws, generalizations, or associations within particular historical and cultural frameworks for purposes of developing treatment warrants. In the end, there will be concepts, as opposed to a concept, of gender-specific disease.

An integrative account of gender-specific disease carries ethical implications. It carries ethical implications because our understanding of gender-specific disease is evaluative, and some of our evaluations of gender-specific disease entail judgments concerning the praiseworthiness and blameworthiness of the clinical event. To begin with, an integrative understanding of gender-specific disease leads us to rethink the approach we use in bioethics to assess the ethicality of gendering disease. Given the current popularity of a gender-neutral principle-based approach in bioethics, we are encouraged to consider whether a gender-neutral approach is sufficiently able to evaluate a gender-inclusive clinical matter. I argue that it is not sufficient, and that we benefit from adopting a gender-inclusive approach to assessing the ethicality of how we classify and describe gender-specific disease. Of course this makes sense—why would one assess a gender matter with a gender-neutral methodology? Nevertheless, we need to be cautious here. A gender-inclusive bioethical approach must be integrative in order to assess the integrative character of gender, disease, and their relations. If it is not, we risk reducing gender, disease, and their relation to concepts that are either non-contextual or open to the whims of the interpreter. Further, an integrative understanding of gender-specific disease highlights some prominent ethical or normative challenges in framing gender-specific disease. In the end, I am supportive of a "both/and" emphasis on context and integration in relation to both considerations of gender-specific disease and related bioethical analyses.

Indeed, the reader will find that this analysis rehearses ground already covered. There is a significant body of literature in the philosophy of medicine on concepts of disease (Faber 1923; King 1954; Margolis 1976; Sontag 1978; Reznek 1987; Caplan et al. 1981; Humber and Almeder 1997; Engelhardt and Wildes 2003; Cutter 2003; Caplan et al. 2004; Murphy 2008). There is a large volume of literature on gender and health (Sherwin 1992; Dreger 1998; Ratcliff 2002; Young 2005; Schulz and Mullings 2006; Bird and Rieker 2008; Mikkola 2008). The extended arguments that gender matters in health care and that culturally entrenched views of women can negatively impact women's health have been made many times over, continuing today with recent texts like the edited collection from the International Association of Feminist Approaches to Bioethics (2011). The need to consider how medicine frames AIDS (Cutter 1989, 1990, 2003; Treichler 1999; Sontag 1989; Shilts 1987), heart disease (Dresser 1992; Legato 2004a), and menopause (Seaman 2003; McCrea 2004) is not a new message. The notion of an integrative approach to disease is the subject of attention on the part of a growing number of clinical practitioners today (e.g., Weil 1995, 2004; Northrup 2002; Kligler and Lee 2004). There is no shortage of discussions in the current feminist bioethical literature about the need to involve discussion of gender in traditional bioethical approaches (Cutter 1992, 1997, 2006; Donchin 2009; Tong 1997, 2004, 2007; Holmes and Purdy 1992; Wolf 1996; Sherwin 1992, 2008; Mahowald 1993; Rawlinson 2001).

Although such discussions are not represented here as new, they are brought together in a single volume to illustrate the integral connectedness among concerns about how medicine genders disease for purposes of providing guidance to those involved in explaining and treating gender-specific disease. For sure there are extended discussions of concepts of disease in the philosophy of medicine literature, but currently there is no sustained discussion of the philosophical nature of *gender-specific* disease. There is overwhelming support in the medical literature that gender matters in disease. Yet, there is a lack of philosophical analysis about how it matters. There are discussions about changes in our medical thinking about AIDS, heart disease, and menopause, but what do these discussions teach us about how medicine genders disease? There are rich discussions of the need for allopathic medicine to adopt a more integrative approach to disease, but how can these discussions help us think through the character of gender-specific disease? There is a huge body of literature in contemporary bioethics, but how are our bioethical approaches extensions of our epistemological commitments? There is a significant body of literature in "feminist bioethics," but how do these discussions guide us in addressing specific ethical issues raised by gendering disease? How do our reflections on gendering disease shed light on how we ought to proceed in our bioethical analyses?

In addition to the benefits, what might be the harms of an integrative gender-specific approach to disease? To what extent does the recognition of pluralism in ontological, epistemological, axiological, and bioethical discussions of gender-specific disease risk relativism and the undermining of useful and reliable gender-specific descriptions and prescriptions? To what extent do the simultaneous critique and defense of partiality in philosophical discourse on gender matters in medicine risk illogical thinking and the undermining of current practices in medicine? To what extent does the recognition that gender matters in disease risk "gender imperialism," the view that all diseases are best conceptualized as gender-specific diseases? To what extent does the recognition that gender matters in disease risk "gender contagion," the view that "my gender caused my disease" or "my gender made me sick"? These and related benefits and challenges raised by this project will be considered.

As a working mother, I could not have engaged in this project without the great support of others. I thank reviewers for their helpful comments and their encouragement to take further the topics that I raise. In particular, I thank Mark Cherry for the time spent discussing the project and for his insightful suggestions on how to improve it. This final project may be far from what reviewers envisioned, but I can assure them that their comments have led me to pursue this project with greater focus. I continue to be grateful to H. Tristram Engelhardt, Jr., for sharing many years ago his expertise in philosophy of medicine, and in particular his interest in the philosophical issues raised by nosologies and nosographies. I am grateful to my administrators and colleagues at the University of Colorado at Colorado Springs for their continued support of my work in philosophy of medicine, bioethics, and applied ethics. I am particularly indebted to Raphael Sassower and Fred Bender for their collaborations, discussions, and encouragement over these many years. I am grateful as well to Dorothea Olkowski, Rex Welshon, Sonja Tanner, Lorraine Arangno, Mary Jane Sullivan, Teresa Meadows, Rebecca Laroche, and Tom Christensen for their guidance and willingness to step into my shoes in offering it. My friends in the beautiful Rocky Mountain town of Steamboat Springs, Colorado, have shown me that it indeed takes a village to raise a family. Betsy Johnston, Sophie Melvin, Laurie Hall, Lisa-Marie Baker, and Al Weisberg—thanks for looking out for Lewis, Theresa, and John during my absences. Anne Sarno, Laura Sansone, and my students have continued to be inspirations as I work at the desk, on the computer, and in the classroom. A most special indebtedness goes to my husband, Lew, for putting up with an academic who is nagged by the logical contradictions of life. Thanks for protecting and honoring my reading, writing, and traveling time—but moreover, thank you for your unconditional support; I know now that the unconditional is philosophically and humanly possible. Last, but not least, thank you to my father, John P. Gardell, and his wife Vera, and my mother M. Theresa Gardell, who have remained beacons of wisdom and uncompromising supporters of education all these years. This work on women is dedicated to my father, John, a guy who knew well before the popularity of second-wave feminism that women deserved better. Your encouragement has made projects like this possible. For this, I remain indebted to you.

Colorado Springs and Steamboat Springs, Colorado
July 23, 2011

1 Background

INTRODUCTION

This chapter introduces the reader to a philosophical study of the ethics of gender-specific disease. It rehearses key discussions about gender-specific medicine, disease, gender and sex, and women that emerge in this inquiry. It closes with a brief overview of the organization of the study.

WHY STUDY GENDER-SPECIFIC MEDICINE?

Gender-specific, or as some call it sex-specific, medicine is heralded as a "new field of medicine" (Weisfeldt 2004, xiii) and a "new science" (Legato 2004b, xv). It emerges in the late twentieth century as a response to the need to investigate "gender as an important variable [of disease manifestation and treatment] in our research protocols" (Legato 2004b, xv). It studies "the unique aspects of men's biology as it is to that of women" (Legato 2010b, xxi). There is increased evidence for gender and sex differences in, for instance, coronary artery disease, cardiovascular disease, addiction times, drug metabolism, carcinogenic effects of tobacco smoke, risk of lung cancer, differential HIV viral load and treatment options, and depression (Legato 2004c, 2010b; also see Institute of Medicine 2001a, 2001b; Nobelius and Wainer 2004). There is little disagreement that, among women and men, some diseases have different frequencies (e.g., in the case of lupus, heart disease, and depression), different symptoms (e.g., in the case of acute myocardial infarction, gonorrhea, and AIDS), different diagnoses (e.g., in the case of acute myocardial infarction and AIDS), different prognoses (e.g., in the case of AIDS, heart disease, and lung cancer), and different treatments (e.g., in the case of AIDS, hypothyroidism, and post-traumatic stress disorder) (for numerous other examples, see Nobelius and Wainer 2004; Legato 2004c; Langley 2004). There is growing agreement in the clinical community that there is a need for "a serious focus on gender as a critical and determining factor in understanding human biology, the nature of human disease, and therapy and management both acutely and chronically" (Weisfeldt 2004, xiii).

As an example, consider cardiology. In 2006, heart disease was the leading cause of mortality for women and men in the U.S. Cardiovascular disease took approximately 315,930 women and 315,706 men that year (Heron 2010, 9). Except for perhaps neurologists (Byrne 2004) and pediatricians (Lazarus 2004), no group of clinicians has given more thought to the impact of gender on the experience of disease than cardiologists (Legato 2004a, 183). Physician Jonathan Tobin et al.'s landmark article (1987) brought to cardiologists' attention differences in the ways cardiologists responded to the complaints of women and men with coronary heart disease (Legato 2004a, 183). A number of research studies in the twentieth century investigating heart disease included only men as research subjects, even though the results concerning the diagnosis of heart disease were applied to women (Dresser 1992). Research showed that women are more likely to exhibit symptoms like shortness of breath and fatigue as indicators of a heart attack compared to men who usually experience the classic chest pain. Today, there has been a large body of literature noting gender-specific differences in normal myocardial anatomy and physiology and in the experience of diseases of the cardiovascular system (Legato and Legha 2004), the different quantitative impact of risk factors for coronary artery disease on women and men (Bassuk and Manson 2004), different features of its clinical course (Roberts 2004), and difference responses to therapeutics (Rosen and Pham 2004).

The past few decades have witnessed significant growth in gender-specific medicine. In 1997, the physician, cardiologist, and researcher Marianne J. Legato founded the Partnership for Women's Health (2007) at Columbia University in New York City, New York. This partnership was the first of its kind between an academic medical center and the private sector that focused solely on gender-specific medicine. The center, which has since changed its name to the Partnership for Gender-Specific Medicine (Partnership for Gender-Specific Medicine 2008), is responsible for the publication of the *Journal of Gender-Specific Medicine* (2008), or as it is called today *Gender Medicine* (2011). Since then, a number of medical schools have formed programs in gender-specific medicine (Henrich and Viscoli 2006; Glezerman 2010), although many are still marginalized in the large medical centers and there is not yet available a board-certified specialty in the field. The seminal two-volume set entitled *The Principles of Gender-Specific Medicine* (Legato 2004c) appeared in 2004 and features fourteen areas of study of clinical differences between women and men, including development, central nervous system, cardiology, pulmonology, gastroenterology, reproductive biology, oncology, nutrition, drug metabolism, infectious disease, immunology, rheumatology, aging, and dermatology. A second edition appeared in 2010 (Legato 2010b) and focuses on the essentials of gender-specific disease.

In 1999, the Institute of Medicine, the health arm of the National Academy of Sciences, formed the Committee on Understanding the Biology of Sex and Gender Differences to attend to cataloguing the knowledge on and research priorities for animal and cellular models that could be used to determine when sex and gender differences exist and when they are relevant to biologic functioning at the cellular, physiological, anatomical, developmental, and behavioral levels. In addition, it set out to identify current and potential barriers to the conduct of valid and productive research on sex and gender differences and their determinants, including ethical, financial, sociological, and scientific. It sought to define strategies that can be used to overcome such barriers and promote the acceptance of this research by the scientific community and general public (Moncher and Douglas 2004, 279). In 2001, the Institute of Medicine published its findings in a report entitled *Exploring the Biological Contributions to Human Health: Does Sex Matter?* (2001a) and provided evidence in support of a biological basis of sex differences in health and disease. *Exploring* distinguishes between biological sex differences and socially acquired gender differences, reviews evidence for the contribution of biological sex to women's and men's health, and calls for an evaluation of the contribution of sex in all biological and health research. In 2001 as well, the Institute of Medicine published *Health and Behavior: The Interplay of Biological, Behavioral, and Social Influences* (2001b). *Health* examines the link between health and behavior, the influence of psychological factors or behavior, and the benefits of intervening at different levels to improve individual and population health.

In the Preface to *The Principles of Gender-Specific Medicine,* Legato defines "gender-specific medicine" as the "study of the differences in men and women's normal function and in their experience of the same diseases" (Legato 2004b, xv). In the 2010 edition, she defines "gender-specific medicine" as the "study of how the normal function and the experience of disease differs between men and women" (Legato 2010a, xxi). The Partnership for Women's Health at Columbia University similarly defines gender-specific medicine as "the science of how normal human biology differs between men and women and how the manifestation, mechanisms, and treatment of disease vary as a function of gender" (Partnership for Women's Health 2007). One might note that the definitions above share the view that gender-specific medicine attends to how "normal" biological "function" or biology "differs" between the "genders" in the "same" disease, thus highlighting key claims in our understanding of gender-specific disease.

The forthcoming analysis submits the notion of gender-specific disease to philosophical scrutiny. It attends to the meaning of "normal" and "function" and asks whether a biomedical understanding of such notions can adequately account for what is being addressed and treated in gender-specific disease. It considers the challenge of determining "difference" between women and men, and females and males, and asks whether these differences based on biomedical criteria are sufficient to account for what is being investigated. It explores how "gender" and "disease" are understood in gender-specific medicine and how gender is understood as a causal "variable" in disease expression and treatment. Legato herself highlights this central challenge concerning the causal relation between gender and disease when she asks: "[H]ow much . . . of being 'male' and 'female' is hardwired into us from conception and evolves inevitably—and how much is plastic, mutable and dependent on where and how we exist? . . . What's the consequence of biologic sex and what's essentially a result of gender [in disease manifestation and treatment]?" (Legato 2004b, xv–xvi). This inquiry hopes to aid in addressing Legato's query as it maps the philosophical terrain of gender-specific disease.

WHY STUDY DISEASE?

Physician-philosopher Edmund D. Pellegrino recently said that "[i]n light of its unquestioned power to affect human life, clarification of medicine's basic concepts is as much a moral as an intellectual obligation. Confusion about the nature of health and disease is ultimately confusion about the concept of medicine itself" (2004, xii). In order to avoid confusion in medical theory and practice, Pellegrino recommends philosophical inquiry into major concepts in medicine. Heeding Pellegrino's suggestions, this inquiry investigates the philosophical terrain of gender-specific disease in order to aid clarification in gender-specific taxonomy and nomenclature.

A study of *disease* is important because disease is a centralizing notion in health care, one that has direct and important consequences for daily life. How medicine classifies, describes, and explains disease guides medical diagnosis and treatment. It guides what actions are advised to be taken and which ones are not, as well as who is charged with what tasks. If one is diagnosed with lung cancer, for instance, there will be certain avenues of treatment (e.g., chemotherapy) that will be recommended. If one is diagnosed with congestive heart failure, one would not receive treatments recommended for lung cancer but rather receive some other kind of intervention (e.g., minimally invasive heart surgery). For the most part, what one is diagnosed with guides treatment, and what one is treated with reflects what one is diagnosed with.

Further, how medicine classifies, describes, and explains disease evokes the allocation of vast amounts of societal and personal resources. In 2009, the U.S. spent 17.6% of its Gross Domestic Product (GDP) on health care, a figure that translates into $2.5 trillion dollars. In the U.S., Medicare spent 20% of the total of national health expenditure, resulting in $502.8 billion dollars and Medicaid spent 15% of the total of national health expenditure, resulting in $373.9 billion dollars. Private spending constituted 32% of the total national health expenditure, resulting in $801.2 billion dollars. The federal government's share of health care spending increased just over three percentage points in 2009 to 27%, whereas the share of spending by households (28%), and state and local governments (16%) fell by one percentage point each (Department of Health and Human Services 2010).

Another reason to study disease is to appreciate our historical past (see, e.g., Faber 1923; Garrison 1929; King 1963, 1984; Kraupl-Taylor 1979) and gain insight into directions for future developments. How we understand disease today is a reflection of our past ways of knowing. Eighteenth-century clinician and botanist Carolus Linnaeus (1707–1778) developed a taxonomy of disease that included eleven classes of disease based on clinical signs and symptoms. These included *exanthematici* (e.g., smallpox), *critici* (i.e., critical fevers), *phlogistici* (i.e., inflammations), *dolorosi* (i.e., painful diseases), *mentales* (i.e., mental disturbances), *quietales* (i.e., impairment of voluntary actions), *motorii* (i.e., convulsive diseases), *suppressorii* (i.e., suppression of bodily fluids), *evacuatorii* (i.e., discharge of fluid), *deformes* (i.e., physical wasting), and *vitia* (i.e., skin diseases) (Linnaeus, translated in Bowman 1976, 9). These eleven classes of disease reflect how clinicians classified the clinical complaints patients brought to the clinic. Not knowing about viruses, Linnaeus classified rabies as a mental disturbance, and not knowing about vitamin deficiency, he classified rickets as physical wasting (Bowman 1976). Early taxonomies reflect a way to organize patient signs and symptoms into categories that were useful for diagnosis.

In contrast to Linnaeus, in the nineteenth century, cellular pathologist Rudolf Virchow (1821–1902) began to classify disease in terms of anatomic and physiological underpinnings. The early Virchow understood diseases not as "self-subsistent, self-contained entities" (1981 [1858], 188) or invading organisms, but as states indicative of underlying pathophysiological processes. Disease represented "only the course of corporeal appearances under changed conditions" (1981 [1858], 188). For the early Virchow, disease should not be confused with its causes: "Scientific medicine has as its object the discovery of changed conditions, characterizing the sick body or the individual suffering organ. Its object is also the delineation of deviations experienced by the phenomena of life under certain conditions" (1981 [1858], 188). Disease is understood in terms of its pathophysiological processes as deviations from normal bodily conditions, as opposed to patient signs and symptoms.

The transformation of clinical classifications from an enterprise that catalogued patient symptoms to one that organized anatomic and physiological observations and measurements allowed a reorganization of clinical classifications and the diagnoses and treatments that followed. Conditions such as fever and pain were no longer considered diseases in their own right, but symptoms associated with underlying physiological processes that were in turn given a name (e.g., tuberculosis, malaria). Previously discriminated problems (e.g., coughing up blood, shortness of breath) could now be brought together under the same rubric (e.g., tuberculosis). Clinical complaints that had not been discriminated (e.g., pain) could now be distinguished in terms of their anatomical and physiological locations (e.g., hernia, arthritis). These changes in clinical classifications led to the notion that the goals of medicine are not found in the mere reporting of patient signs and symptoms, but rather in comprehending the pathophysiological processes of such reportings (Engelhardt 1982; Foucault 1973 [1963]). Today, it is no wonder that medicine assigns the laboratory a central role in clinical medicine and relies heavily on laboratory tests as opposed to clinical reporting in determining why a patient is ill.

Anatomical and physiological specialties have grown and the number of taxonomies employed by clinicians far exceeds the eleven offered by Linnaeus. The International Classification of Disease, 10th edition (ICD-10) used today contains approximately twelve thousand categories of disease and serves numerous health care purposes. Disease nosologies no longer involve simple classifications of symptoms and internal pathophysiological processes. They detail a host of ways to explain clinical events defined by:

1. *symptomatology—manifestations*: known pattern of signs, symptoms, and related findings
2. *etiology*: an underlying explanatory mechanism
3. *course and outcome*: a distinct pattern of development over time
4. *treatment response*: a known pattern of response to interventions
5. *linkage to genetic factors*: e.g., genotypes, patterns of gene expression
6. *linkage to interacting environmental factors* (Production of ICD-11: The Revision Process 2007)

Disease entries in ICD-10 are used for numerous purposes, including the analysis of the general health situation of population groups and monitoring of the incidence and prevalence of diseases and other health problems in relation to other variables, such as the characteristics and circumstances of the individuals affected, reimbursement, resource allocation, quality, and guidelines. They are used internationally to classify diseases and other health problems recorded on many types of health and vital records, including death certificates and health records. In addition to enabling the storage and retrieval of diagnostic information for clinical, epidemiological, and quality purposes, they also provide the basis for the compilation of national mortality and morbidity statistics by World Health Organization (WHO) Member States (World Health Organization 1992). The next version of the ICD (11th edition) is due out in 2015 and is expected to have more than twelve thousand taxonomies of disease (Production of ICD-11: The Revision Process 2007).

In addition to disease being a centralizing notion in medicine, a reason to allocate resources, and a window into the roots of our past, disease is a term that calls out for clarification. There is a sense in which disease and health are related (Engelhardt and Wildes 2003; Murphy 2008). Indeed, health often refers to the absence of disease or illness in situations where the individual does not have a disease, as might be in cases of *not* having a positive test for tuberculosis or carcinoma of the lung. On this view, either one has a disease or one does not. Yet, as one can well imagine, health may

WHY STUDY GENDER AND SEX?

This inquiry focuses as well on *gender or sex* as "an important variable [of disease manifestation and treatment] in our research protocols" (Legato 2004b, xv). Perhaps a brief background (Mikkola 2008) on the terms "gender" and "sex" provides a sense of the complexity of the challenge of determining "[w]hat's the consequence of biologic sex and what's essentially a result of gender [in disease manifestation and treatment]?" (Legato 2004b, xv–xvi). Typically in medicine, "sex" is a term used by clinicians to refer to the biological and physiological features that define what it means to be "female" and "male" (Hyde and Whipple 2005, 171; World Health Organization 2010). Identification of sex is based on certain key biological factors such as genital structure (e.g., clitoris, penis), hormonal make-up (e.g., estrogen progesterone, testosterone), and genetic (chromosomal) patterns (e.g., XX, XY) (Hyde and Whipple 2005, 173–74). Increasingly it refers to the "genotype," the XX and XY, that defines "female" and "male," respectively. In contrast, "gender" is typically used by clinicians to refer "to the socially constructed roles, behaviours, activities, and attributes that a given society considers appropriate for men and women" (World Health Organization 2010). It is the "phenotype" that results from embedding a female or male in her or his culture, and is typically referred to as woman and girl, or man and boy, respectively.

According to feminist philosopher Iris Marion Young (2005), the sex-gender distinction gained notoriety in the mid-twentieth century with the rise of second-wave feminism, the mid- to late-twentieth-century movement that sought equality between the sexes. In the 1970s, it has served the purpose of conceptualizing capacities and dispositions of members of both sexes that distanced behavior, temperament, and achievement from biological or natural explanations. Feminists and others could affirm that women and men are different in physical and reproductive functions, while denying that these differences have any relevance for the opportunities members of the sexes should have or the activities in which they should engage. Much of this early second-wave feminist theorizing invoked an ideal of equality for women that envisioned an end to gender. With this change, as Young puts it, "[w]e would all be just people with various bodies" (2005, 13).

Support for the sex-gender distinction came under fire with feminists working in the late 1970s and early 1980s (Young 2005). Feminist philosopher Nancy Chodorow (1978), feminist psychologist Carol Gilligan (1982), and feminist social scientist Nancy Hartsock (1983, 1998) developed accounts of the social and psychological specificities of femininely gendered identity and social perspective derived from gender roles. Chodorow analyzed the development of stereotypical feminine and masculine traits in terms of the different problems of identity-formation by female and male children who are raised by female caretakers. Gilligan explored feminine moral epistemologies that emphasize relatedness and affect to counterbalance the traditional (male) emphasis on understanding moral reasoning as a process that takes the reasoner from a moral principle to a particular moral judgment. Hartsock was concerned with the development of theory in response to current feminist concerns and within feminist communities dealing with representation and social change and recommended greater efforts to include marginalized voices in discussions. Together these thinkers focus on accounts of feminine gender identities as expressing a social standpoint defining the lives and possibilities of women and subsequent actions that are necessary and appropriate to stimulate social change.

These views of feminine identities were met with sharp criticism. Many, and especially Gilligan (1982) in the general literature, were attacked for offering "essentialist" or "realist" accounts of women, the view that all women are of a certain kind or nature based on some essential feature. Gilligan was seen to characterize women in compartmentalized categories and to support certain stereotypes or harmful generalizations of women as, for example, mothers, caretakers, and compromisers. She was critiqued for failing to take into consideration significant dimensions of difference (e.g., race and class positioning) in women's lives and the effects these have in differentiating women's experiences and challenges. Gilligan became identified with Anglo, middle-class politics, lifestyles, and sexuality.

According to Young (2005), the need for an account of gender identity that breaks from "gender essentialism" or "gender realism" came notably from feminist philosopher Judith Butler in *Gender Trouble* (1990). Butler cautioned that the feminist distinction between sex and gender retains a binarism of stable categorical complementarity between female and male which produces a logic of normativity, such as the norm of the "ideal" female and male, the norm of a certain relation between a female and male, and the norm of social performance for females and males. In *Bodies That Matter* (1993), Butler argued that the materiality of sexed bodies is itself socially constituted. How the body is seen, categorized, portrayed, celebrated, and lamented relies on social contexts. As she puts it, "the regulatory norms of 'sex' work in a performative fashion to constitute the materiality of bodies and, more specifically, to materialize the body's sex, to materialize sexual difference in the service of the consolidation of the heterosexual imperative" (1993, 2). In other words, gender pressures to conform lead to actual changes in the material or biological structure of sex for purposes of achieving certain social goals. In the end, Butler successfully called into question the logic of the sex-gender distinction.

For an alternative to the categories of sex and gender, philosopher Toril Moi (2001) proposed to return to the framework of Continental Existential Phenomenology on which philosopher Simone de Beauvoir relies. As de Beauvoir famously said, "[o]ne is not born, but rather becomes, a woman. No biological, psychological, or economic fate determines the figure that the human female presents in society; it is our civilization as a whole that produces this creature" (1952, xxxiv). The central category for this theoretical approach is that of the *lived body*. A reconstituted concept of the lived body would offer feminists an idea that could serve the function feminists had wanted from the sex-gender categorization, but without the problems. According to Moi, the lived body is a unified idea of a physical body acting and experiencing in a specific socio-cultural context. It is the body composed of organs, tissues, and cells of a certain size, age, health, and training in relation to its socio-historical environment composed of food, shelter, climate, geography, politics, and, I would add, health care. It resists categorization dimorphically, biologically, and in terms of identity politics. By means of a category of the lived body, then, "one can arrive at a highly historicized and concrete understanding of bodies and subjectivity without relying on the sex-gender distinction" (Moi 2001, 46).

But, as Young (2005) points out, the challenge with Moi's view in feminism within the walls of medicine is to resist reducing women to her subjectivity. Not only is this another form of essentialism, of stereotyping women as psychological beings of a certain kind, but this may not help in allowing us to critique a socio-political system such as medicine for the ways in which it generalizes about women, bodies, and disease. According to Young, we may still need a concept of gender to be able to describe the rules and practices of institutions that grant differing roles for women and men and for understanding how and why certain patterns in the allocation of tasks or status recognition remain persistent in ways that limit opportunities for women. As Young puts it, "I want to suggest that a concept of gender [in medicine] is important for theorizing social structures and their implication for the freedom and well being of persons" (2005, 19).

The analysis that follows heeds Young's advice and retains the categories of gender and sex in the context of gender-specific medicine. In keeping with the use of the terms in medicine (with exceptions that are evident in the literature), it employs (at least initially) the language of "woman" and "man" to refer to the so-called "social construction of sex" and the language of "female" and "male" to designate the so-called "biological description of gender." It employs the term "*gender*-specific disease" in keeping with how it is used in the contemporary clinical literature. It explores the meaning and use of such terms against the backdrop of clinical, philosophical, sociological, and feminist analyses of how gender and sex is understood in gender-specific medicine. It calls into question the possibility of arriving at an unequivocal unambiguous sociological account of gender and biological account of sex, as well as a binary account of woman and man, and female and male. It further calls into question an account of gender-specific or sex-specific factors as single causal variables in disease expression. At the same time, it eschews the relativist standpoint that it is impossible to say anything in clinical medicine about gender and sex and their relation to disease. A reconception of how gender and sex are understood in gender-specific disease serves to assist gender-specific medicine in moving beyond problematic ways of understanding and treating gender-specific disease in women's health care.

WHY FOCUS ON WOMEN?

Most of the examples of gender-specific disease presented in this analysis are drawn from women's health care. This is not to suggest that gender-specific medicine is women's health care or that there is nothing that needs to be said about health care offered to those other than women (Glezerman 2010, xviii). A study of women's disease as a major case study of gender-specific disease allows us to focus this work and consider some pressing needs in women's health care. Although I offer a brief discussion of the implications of the conclusions of this study for health care for men, children, and members of the lesbian, gay, transgender, and bisexual communities, subsequent projects would serve patients well by taking up the question of how medicine can best serve particular gender-specific medical needs.

In addition to focusing this work, there are a number of reasons to study gender-specific disease in the context of women's health care. Almost two-thirds of the diseases that affect both females and males have been studied exclusively in men (DeLorey 2007). This is the case in part because medicine has traditionally excluded women from medical research because of concerns about hazards and risks of clinical interventions on a potentially-child-bearing woman, a pregnant woman, and any potential or actual fetus (Dresser 1992). Yet, women make up 52% of the U.S. population and generally use the health care system more frequently than do men. Women have greater annual health care expenses than men ($2,453 vs. $2,316) and pay a greater proportion of their health care expenses out-of-pocket (19% vs. 16%). Women make 58% more visits each year to primary care physicians and are more likely than men to take at least one prescription drug on a daily basis (DeLorey 2007). Because women typically live longer (Centers for Disease Control and Prevention 2006), they use health care services longer than men.

Further, as is well documented, medicine has a tradition of viewing women in a way that has been the focus of vocal criticism (Tuana 1988; Tavris 1992). What follows entails some of the highlights of this history. Most have heard the stories of how the Ancient Greek philosopher Aristotle (384–322 B.C.E.), the son of a physician, thought women were "deformed." According to Aristotle, the female was "a sort of natural deficiency" of "heat" because she had "a smaller portion" of it (*The generation of animals*, 1984, 726.b.33). The male "semen" was the result of an infusion of heat that concentrated the potency of blood and changed its appearance. Women were unable to "cook" their semen to the point of purity, and thus were "cold," resulting in red (menstruation) as opposed to white reproductive seed (*The generation of animals* 1984, 726.b.30–31). Further,

Aristotle granted a special role to the male in procreation. "By definition the male is that which is able to generate in another . . . the female is that which is able to generate in itself and out of which comes into being the offspring previously existing in the generator" (*The generation of animals* 1984, 716.1.20–23). Here Aristotle did not hold the view that the male introduced the full offspring into the female, a view offered in 1694 by Dutch physicist Nicolaus Hartsoeker (1856–1725) (*Essai de diotropique,* in Tuana 1988, 54). Rather, he held the view that the male imparted the *form* of the fetus into the female and the female's role was to provide the *material,* the menstrual blood, upon which the male semen imparted the form (Tuana 1988, 38). An early view of female bodily inferiority is established in biology and medicine.

Following in the footsteps of Aristotle, the Ancient Greek physician Galen of Pergamum (129–200/217 A.D.) offered a view of female bodily inferiority. The female, he said, was "less perfect than the male" (1968, 14.II.295). Women's genitals "were formed within her when she was still a fetus" (Galen 1968, 14.II.299), but could not develop because of a defect in the heat in a female's body. It is for this reason that a woman's genitals appeared outside in (Laqueur 1990, 25). Having established the imperfection of women's genitals, Galen proceeded to claim that women's semen was similarly imperfect. "[T]he female must have smaller, less perfect testes, and the semen generated in them must be scantier, colder, and wetter" (Galen 1968, 14.II.301). As with Aristotle, Galen blamed the source of woman's defect on her lack of "heat" in the left testis (ovary) as a consequence of limited nourishment, compared to the right testis (ovary), a position handed down from the Ancient Greek physician Hippocrates (1943 [fifth c. B.C.E.], XXVII & XXIX] and perpetuated by a host of others (e.g., Vesalius 1950, Plate 61 from *De Humani Corporis Fabrica,* in Tuana 1988) in anatomical sketches to support their claims.

This hegemony of the primacy of the male generative powers and the inferiority of the female body continued well into medieval and modern medicine. The views of Aristotle and Galen found expression in the works of anatomist Ricardi Anglici (1180–1225), Albertus Magnis (1206–1280), Andres de Laguna (1499–1560), Niccolo Massa (1485–1569), and Hermann Boerhaave (1668–1738) (Tuana 1988, 47–51), all of whom came up with creative anatomical findings to account for the inferiority of the female generative power. There were a number of accounts here, including the view that the female was divinely inspired to be different. Another popular theory, known as the "epigenetic theory of development" (Tuana 1988, 51), promoted the view that the fetus resulted from the gradual development of unorganized matter from the female and the organizing form or force from the male. On this account, the female made some contribution to reproduction, but her role was subordinate to the male offering.

Nineteenth-century clinical medicine echoes the view that woman's bodies were different and difference is deficit. The difference has to do with the female reproductive system. As Dr. Dirix put it in 1856, "[t]hese diseases [of women] will be found, on due investigation, to be in reality, no disease at all, but merely the sympathetic reaction or the symptoms of one disease, a disease of the womb" (quoted in Smith-Rosenberg and Rosenberg 1981, 284). Dr. Holbrook said it this way in 1882: "[I]t was as if the Almighty, in creating the female sex, had taken the uterus and built up a woman around it" (quoted in Smith-Rosenberg and Rosenberg 1981, 284). In 1893, Dr. Rohe analyzed "lactational insanity" (i.e., depression) at the forty-fourth Annual Meeting of the American Medical Society in this way: "Prolonged or excessive lactation is given as the chief cause of [insanity (i.e., depression)]. . . . In most cases, this is probably true, yet there are some cases in which the disease must be attributed to other etiological factors. . . . It appears . . . that the local [i.e., pelvic] irritations acting upon the central organ [i.e., the brain] are active, both as determining the duration as well as the course of the mental disorder" (quoted in Weissman and Olfson 1995, 799).

In the twentieth century, the reproductive roots of women's disease dominated clinicians' attention. In 1966, gynecologist Robert A. Wilson gained public notoriety with the publication of his best seller, *Feminine Forever* (1966). In it, he explained the plight of menopausal women and offered the cure for their "deficiency disease," which he compared with diabetes (Wilson 1966, 18; Houck 2006, 156). He claimed that estrogen therapy actually served nature's plan by maintaining the necessary hormonal balance. "The prematurely aging castrate," rather than the medically restored woman, was "unnatural" (Wilson 1966, 53; Houck 2006, 156–57). For Wilson, estrogen was the answer: "Estrogen therapy is a proven, effective means of restoring the normal balance of her bodily and psychic functions throughout her prolonged life. It is nothing less than the method by which a woman can remain *feminine forever*" (Wilson 1966, 54, *my italics*). Estrogen, he wrote, "aside from keeping a woman sexually attractive and potent . . . preserves the strength of her bones, the glow of her skin, the gloss of her hair. . . . Estrogen makes women adaptable, even tempered, and generally easy to live with" (Wilson 1966, 62, 64). Wilson encouraged women to see themselves as having a duty to reverse their dwindling estrogen levels: "If the question is to be examined on philosophic grounds, I rest my case on the simple contention that castration is a bad thing and that every woman has the right— indeed the duty—to counteract castration that befalls her during her middle years" (Wilson 1966, 54). Wilson promised much with estrogen therapy; he repeated his notion that estrogen prevents breast and endometrial cancer and cures unwanted symptoms, citing his own *Journal of the American Medical Association* article (1962) (Wilson 1966, 67). His view carried much influence well into the late twentieth century, resulting in a significant rise in the use of hormone therapy among women (Hersh et al. 2004).

The rise of what many call the "women's health movement" (Ruzek and Becker 1998) in the U.S. in the 1970s is in part a response to a history of marginalizing woman in medicine. It is a result of a complex set of forces, including developments in public awareness, clinical practice, clinical research, and health policies. Issues raised by advocates of the rights of women and minorities, consumers, the mentally ill, and prisoners in the 1970s often included health care components and helped reinforce public acceptance of women's concerns regarding their health care. The women's health movement in particular encouraged and continues to encourage women to question established medical authority (Federation of Feminist Women's Health Centers 1981; National Women's Health Network 2009), to take responsibility for their own bodies (Boston Women's Health Book Collective 1973, 1998; Worcester and Whatley 2005), and to express new demands for clinical research and access to appropriate health care (Dresser 1996; Merton 1996; Purdy 1996; Moncher and Douglas 2004).

By the mid-1970s, more than 250 formally identifiable women's groups provided education, advocacy, and direct health service in the U.S. (Ruzek 1978, 245–65). Specific concerns of such groups included issues such as endometriosis, breast health, birth control, pregnancy health, childbirth practices, the medicalization of premenstrual syndrome (PMS) and menopause, and the use of diethylstilbestrol (DES). Groups ranged from the formation of the Boston Women's Health Book Collective, the Federation of Feminist Women's Health Centers, the National Women's Health Network, National Black Women's Health Project, the National Latina Women's Health Organization, the Native American Women's Health Education and Resource Center, the National Asian Women's Health Organization, the Dis-Abled Women's Network, the Older Women's League, and the Lesbian Health Agenda (Ruzek and Becker 1998, 23). The Nurses' Health Study, which began in 1976, began to explore the risk factors associated with cancer and cardiovascular disease among women. Given the array of interests and actions, the "women's health movement" might better be thought of as the "women's health movements."

A few health policy initiatives in the U.S. are worth mentioning to highlight significant change in how medicine has viewed women in the twentieth century. In 1985, a Task Force on Women's Health Issues began work to aid the Public Health Service (PHS) to improve the health and well-being of women (Department of Health and Human Services 1985). It claimed to focus on problems in women's health that are not simply reducible to reproductive problems and offered this definition of women's health: "[D]iseases or conditions that are unique to or more prevalent or serious in women, have distinct causes or manifest themselves differently in women, or have different outcomes or interventions" (Department of Health and Human Services 1985). Here difference is just difference, and not (what it had long been interpreted as) deficit. The Task Force vowed to focus on promoting a safe and healthful physical and social environment, providing services for the prevention and treatment of disease, conducting research and evaluation, recruiting and training health care personnel, educating and informing the public, and designing guidance for legislative and regulatory measures.

In 1991, Congress established the Office of Women's Health (OWH) within the U.S. Department of Health and Human Services (DHHS). OWH coordinates all the efforts of DHHS's agencies and offices involved in women's health, such as the National Institutes of Health (NIH), the Food and Drug Administration (FDA), the Centers for Disease Control and Prevention (CDC), and other agencies and departments. Its focus continues to be on health education, health care innovation, health disparities, and policy development (Office of Women's Health 2007). In 1991, as well, the U.S. Congress launched the Women's Health Initiative (WHI), a program of the DHHS, NIH, and National Heart, Lung, and Blood Institute (NHLBL), and the largest project of its kind, seeking data on the prevention and treatment of cardiovascular disease, cancer, and osteoporosis.

In 1993, the NIH issued guidelines to ensure that federally funded investigations include an analysis to determine whether the interventions being studied affect women and members of minority groups differently from other groups. Further, section 429B of the NIH Revitalization Act (U.S. Congress 1993) enjoined the NIH Director to guarantee that women and members of minority groups are included in all research projects, unless exclusion is appropriate because of health, the specific focus of the research, or other circumstances that the NIH Director approves. In 1993 as well, the FDA issued *Guidelines for the Study and Evaluation of Gender Differences in the Clinical Evaluation of Drugs* (1993) and altered a sixteen-year-old policy from 1977 that had excluded most women of child-bearing potential from the early phases of clinical trials. Reasons cited for excluding women included women's fluctuations in hormone levels and greater difficulty in getting women to sign up for research projects because they had domestic responsibilities (Moncher and Douglas 2004). Guidelines state that scientists must formulate research hypotheses so as not to exclude sex as a crucial part of the research investigation. For example, when exploring the metabolism of a particular drug, one must routinely run tests on both females and males in order to ensure that potential differences in drug reaction and efficacy between the sexes are analyzed. In 1993, the DHHS set out to study women's health and how it was addressed in medical education. DHHS studied medical school curricula and recommended changes to include educational sequences in women's health care (Council on Graduate Medical Education 1996).

1997 marks an important year in women's health care. The WHI began a study to address the most common causes of death, disability, and impaired quality of life in post-menopausal women. Launched by the first woman director of the National Institutes of Health, physician Bernadine Healy (who passed in 2011), the WHI involved approximately 161,808 post-menopausal women and planned to study the prevention and causes of heart disease, breast and colon cancer, and osteoporosis. After observing more than sixteen thousand post-menopausal women for roughly five years, in 2002 researchers found conclusively that Prempro, a popular hormone therapy containing a combination of estrogens and progestin, raises the risks of heart attack, stroke, blood clots, and breast cancer. The federally sponsored study of the combination estrogen-progestin hormone treatment was supposed to run for eight years, but the five-year results were so decisive that researchers cut the study short in 2002 and urged participants to stop taking Prempro (Cowley and Springen 2002, 38–39; Women Health Initiative 2007). Since then, WHI researchers have reported that hormone replacement therapy (HRT), or what today is called hormone therapy (HT), does not appear to prevent Alzheimer's disease in older women and that calcium and vitamin D supplements do not protect against colon cancer and osteoporosis at the rates previously thought (Tonnessen 2006, 9).

Granted, the late twentieth century has witnessed significant advances in women's health care, but it does not follow that all problems have been solved. According to medical sociologists Chloe Bird and Patricia Rieker, the WHI was not "able to shed light on a broader array of potential risk factors and social determinants of differences and similarities in men's and women's health, ironically leaving an assessment of gender out of the question" (2008, 25). More specifically, "because of the understandable emphasis on biological factors to explain women's health, the WHI does not represent any movement toward integrating social and biomedical models of health and illness and advancing an understanding of the relationship between physical and mental health" (2008, 25). We can say the same about some of the other advancements in women's health. What is needed, according to Bird and Rieker, is "a more integrative research agenda" (2008, 227) in women's health care in particular and gender-specific medicine in general.

The analysis that follows heeds Bird and Rieker's call for continued work on gender-specific disease and health. It takes advantage of a large body of attention given to women's health over the last few decades and pays close attention to the claims and assumptions gender-specific medicine makes about "females" and "women" in the context of discussing diseases that primarily affect them. It calls into question reducing "female" and "woman" to essential kinds that experience the "same" disease in the "same" way. Further, it sides with Bird and Rieker in calling for a more integrative approach to gender-specific disease. In doing so, it questions whether gender, and for that matter sex, can be reduced to a simple biological phenomena that serves as a single variable in disease expressions. This inquiry hopes to aid in continuing a dialogue about the claims and assumptions made about females and women in the context of classifying, describing, and explaining gender-specific disease.

NAVIGATING WHAT FOLLOWS

The analysis that follows argues that gender-specific disease and related bioethical discourses are philosophically *integrative*. To argue this, the

project explores in Chapters 2 through 4 the philosophical nature of gender-specific disease. In particular, it addresses the conceptual claims and
assumptions that frame gender, disease, and the causal relation between
gender-specific factors and disease. Chapter 2 maps out the descriptive
nature of gender, disease and their relation; Chapter 3 the prescriptive character; and Chapter 4 the contextual character. Chapters 5 bridges what
was separated in Chapters 2 through 4 and shows how the descriptive,
prescriptive, and contextual dimensions of gender-specific disease are not
separate and distinct, but rather integrative. In other words, the descriptive, prescriptive, and contextual roles of classifying and describing gender-
specific disease mutually define and situate each other. This is not simply
a theoretical insight, as Chapter 6 shows, but one that carries practical
implications for gender-specific taxonomies and nomenclature, which in
turn have ramifications in clinical practice. Chapters 7 and 8 take up some
salient bioethical implications of rethinking some of the assumptions and
claims about gender-specific disease. Chapter 7 focuses on the need for a
gender-inclusive approach in bioethics in order to assess normative problems raised by the use of gender-specific taxonomies and nomenclature.
Chapter 8 expands the analysis of the need for a gender-inclusive bioethical
approach to include an integrative one that attends to the mutually constitutive factors that constitute gender-specific disease. Chapter 9 shares some
suggestions for future work on gender-specific disease as it applies to men,
children, lesbians, gays, transgenders, and bisexuals. Chapter 10 shares
some general lessons and challenges that may be drawn from this study. In
the end, as Chapter 11 concludes, the project leads us to reflect on the ethics
of framing gender-specific disease for purposes of highlighting how gender-
specific medicine might proceed carefully in describing, explaining, and
providing prescriptions for gender-specific disease for purposes of minimizing some of the normative problems that might arise.

2 Gender-Specific Disease
Descriptive Analysis

DESCRIBING CLINICAL PHENOMENA

This chapter explores how gender-specific disease provides a descriptive account of human biological dysfunction that differs between the genders. It considers the meaning of gender and sex in the context of descriptive discussions of gender-specific disease. Using language commonly found in the philosophy of disease literature, and adopting it to discussions of gender-specific disease, the chapter contrasts a *naturalist* with a *nominalist* account of gender-specific disease. Here the term "naturalist" comes from the Latin word *naturalis*, which means "by birth, pertaining to nature." The term "nominalist" comes from the Latin word *nominalis*, which means "pertaining to a name." Whereas a naturalist or biomedical approach holds that gender-specific disease is a discoverable entity that has independent existence, a nominalist or constructivist one holds that gender-specific disease is a creation, a name for that which is experienced and reported by patients. Because there are limits to both a naturalist and nominalist understanding of gender-specific disease, the chapter argues in favor of what I call a *methodological naturalist* account of gender-specific disease. A methodological naturalist account of gender-specific disease holds that gender-specific disease describes biomedical observations of gender-specific factors as important variables of disease manifestation and treatment explained via etiological laws, generalizations, and associations. On this view, gender-specific disease is in part discovered and in part created. It reflects what we find in the world as well as the names and interpretations we give to such findings.

DISCOVERING GENDER-SPECIFIC DISEASE

Naturalist View of Gender and Sex

We begin the analysis of gender-specific disease with what I call a *naturalist view of gender*. In its report, *Exploring the Biological Contributions to Human Health: Does Sex Matter?* (2001a), the Institute of Medicine defines gender as "[a] person's self-representation as male or female, or how that person is responded to by social institutions based on the individual's gender presentation" (2001a, 17). The World Health Organization similarly defines gender as "the socially constructed roles, behaviours, activities, and attributes that a given society considers appropriate for men and women" (World Health Organization 2010). In *Principles of Gender-Specific Disease*, physician and editor Marianne Legato defines gender as "the phenotype that comes out of embedding a male or female in his or her culture" (2004b, xv). In the Forward to the second edition of *Principles of Gender-Specific Disease*, physician Marek Glezerman defines gender in this way: "To be feminine or to be masculine are characteristics that are defined by the sociological fabric of our environment, the roles we play in a given society, the functions and habits assigned by the society on us, and the expectations which a given society has set for its members" (Glezerman 2010, xviii). On this view, gender refers to "the social construction of sex." It can be defined descriptively and studied using the empirical tools of the natural and social sciences.

Further, the Institute of Medicine states that "gender is rooted in biology" (2001a, 17). This means that gender is based in *sex*. In medicine, sex is understood as a biological phenomenon, a "classification of living things, generally as male or female according to their reproductive organs and functions assigned by chromosomal complement" (Institute of Medicine 2001a, 17; also see World Health Organization 2010; and Sax 2005, 252–53). The Institute of Medicine further states that "[w]ith respect to sex, humans are generally dimorphic. With some exceptions, individuals are either chromosomally XX and developmentally female or chromosomally XY and developmentally male" (Institute of Medicine 2001a, 17). Legato similarly defines sex as "the chromosomal fact of being male or female" (Legato 2004b, xv) and Glezerman says, "maleness and femaleness are chromosomally determined and thus unchangeable" (Glezerman 2010, xviii). This *naturalist account of sex* views sex as something that actually exists in nature, comes in two kinds, and is discoverable through scientific methods.

In twentieth-century medicine, identification of sex has come to be based on certain key biological factors such as genital structure (e.g., clitoris, penis), hormonal make-up (e.g., estrogen, progesterone, testosterone), and genetic (chromosomal) patterns (e.g., XX for females, XY for males) (Hyde and Whipple 2005, 173–74). With the rise of genetic knowledge, the chromosomal description of sex has come to dominate clinical discussions today. The "XY sex-determination system," as it is called, is found in humans, most other mammals, some insects (*Drosophila*), and some plants (*Ginkgo*). In this system, females have two of the same kind of sex chromosome (XX), and are called the "homogametic" sex. Males have two distinct sex chromosomes (XY), and are called the "heterogametic" sex. The XY sex-determination system was first described independently by Nettie Stevens and Edmund Beecher Wilson in 1905 (Kingsland 2007), and since then, molecular biologists have explored a more subtle dosage of genes that interplay with each other rather than function as a simple linear pathway in which genes determine sex.

The line between sex and gender is a source of discussion in gender-specific medicine. The Institute of Medicine (2001a, 18), Legato, and Glezerman encourage careful use of the terms, reserving "sex" for the biological contribution and "gender" for the environmental contribution of reproductive fitness. For instance, color blindness is caused by a gene on the X chromosome and this can be considered a sex-specific or sex-based disease. Melanoma is found typically on the backs of women's legs and on the backs of men and reflects differences in the type of clothing women and men typically wear (American College of Physicians 2001); this can be considered a gender-based disease. The Institute of Medicine itself recognizes the need "to look at sex and gender as part of a single system in which social elements act with biological elements to produce the body" (2001a, 19). It holds that scientific ground will be broken when the "biological questions . . . are posed as a result of an approach that examines how factors outside the body [presumably those that contribute to "gender"] are translated into differences between male and female bodies" (2001a, 19). The point is that carefully distinguishing between gender and sex, and determining the biological basis of differences between the genders and sexes, are goals of gender-specific medicine.

In order to clarify the role of medicine in this area, there are those who hold that the language of gender is best replaced by the language of sex in discussions of gender-specific disease. In reviewing Legato's *Principles of Gender-Specific Disease,* Dr. Virginia M. Miller of the Mayo Clinic College of Medicine raises concerns about the selection of the term "gender" as opposed to "sex" in the field of gender-specific medicine. As she puts it,

> [t]he choice of the "Gender-specific" rather than "Sex-based" medicine for the title is unfortunate in that conventions developed by the Office of Women's Health Research suggest that the term 'gender' be used to describe how an individual perceives their [sic] interaction in the world, while 'sex' is used to define the genotype of XX and XY chromosome. The text addresses sex-based differences (Miller 2005).

Miller's point is that sex (understood as the genotype of XX and XY chromosome) is the basic biological variable that should be considered when designing and analyzing studies in gender-specific biomedical and health-related research. Her view is that there is now sufficient knowledge of the biological, and more specifically genomic, basis of sex differences to validate the scientific study of sex differences in disease expression and to allow the generation of hypotheses. The next step will be to move from the descriptive to the experimental and establish the conditions that must be in place in order to facilitate and to encourage the scientific study of the origins and mechanisms of sex differences in disease expression.

Nevertheless, on a naturalist view of gender and sex, there is agreement that gender and sex are natural phenomena that contribute to important differences in disease expression and treatment. Both are able to be studied using the tools of science. Greater attention to the role of gender and sex in disease can "aid in the accurate measurement and reporting of differences between men and women and help to communicate clearly how the differences apply to biomedical research, patient care, and policy" (Institute of Medicine 2001a, 175–76).

Naturalist View of Disease

Continuing the analysis of gender-specific disease, a *naturalist view of disease* as a phenomenon to be discovered in nature finds wide support in medicine as well. Seventeenth-century physician Thomas Sydenham (1624–1689) (1981 [1676]) argued that nature delivers the structure of disease, which is characterized by recurring, natural, and enduring patterns of signs and symptoms, or as he calls it, "a history of the disease" (1981 [1676], 146). These patterns, for Sydenham, serve as the basis of clinical classifications and should be documented by physicians. Sydenham wrote during a time when physicians were interested in grounding medicine in science and distancing themselves from speculative or biased thought. Sydenham held that nature produces disease in a "uniform and consistent" manner, "so much so, that for the same disease in different persons the symptoms are for the most part the same; and the selfsame phenomena that you would observe in the sickness of a Socrates you would observe in the sickness of a simpleton" (1981 [1676], 148). The task of the clinician, then, is to "discover the real indications" (1981 [1676], 155) of disease, where "real" means that which is found in nature unmitigated by the speculative thought of the observer. Only then can clinicians develop objective clinical nosologies and nosographies.

More recently, contemporary philosopher Christopher Boorse (1975, 1977, 1997) defends the need for a naturalist account of disease in medicine. Boorse defines disease as follows:

1. The *reference class* is a natural class of organisms of uniform functional design; specifically, an age group of a **sex** of a species.
2. A *normal function* of a part or process within members of the reference class is a statistically typical contribution by it to their **individual survival** and **reproduction**. . . .
3. A *disease* is a type of internal state which is either an impairment of **normal functional ability**, i.e., a reduction of one or more functional abilities below typical efficiency, or a limitation on functional ability caused by environmental agents.
4. *Health* is the absence of disease (Boorse 1977, 562, 567, **my bold**; see also Boorse 1997, 7–8).

For Boorse, the reference class relies on uniform design found in an age group of a sex of a species. By "normal functional ability," Boorse means "the readiness of an internal part to perform all its normal functions on typical occasions with at least typical efficiency" (Boorse 1997, 8). On Boorse's account, to call something a disease involves a claim about the abnormal functional ability of some bodily system and how it compromises individual survival and reproduction. In order to distinguish between health and disease, and the normal and the pathological, medicine relies on a reference class and an empirically verifiable account of statistical normality and biological function (Boorse 1997, 8).

A naturalist account of disease, or what psychiatrist George Engel (1981 [1977], 591) calls a biomedical account of disease, "assumes that the language of chemistry and physics will ultimately suffice to explain biological phenomena." It is an objective, value-neutral biological entity open to scientific investigation using an empirical or positivist methodology. That is, disease is seen to be an object that is separate and distinct from the observer and can be known by the observer and verified by other observers using the tools of measurement and quantification. It is to be distinguished from sin, social deviancy, and civil violation, and from the realm of theology, social work, and law. A naturalist account of disease "embraces both reductionism, the philosophic view that complex phenomena are ultimately derived from a single primary principle, and mind-body dualism, the doctrine that separates the mental from the somatic" (Engel 1981 [1977], 591). It is what works in medicine because it offers a reliable way to interpret nature and produces stable clinical categories to be used in clinical diagnosis and treatment.

Naturalist View of Disease Causation

To call something a "gender-specific disease" rests on a causal assessment of sex as a critical and determining factor in disease expression. Determining the causal relation between gender and disease is a complex scientific and philosophical issue. Following philosopher David Magnus (2004, 234), who focuses on determining the cause(s) of genetic disease, I call the problem of determining the causal factors in gender-specific disease "the selection problem." Determining a *naturalistic "causal" relation between gender-specific factors and disease* involves identifying how gender-specific factors bring about a particular disease. There are different ways to talk about causal relation, but for purposes of this analysis, consider at least three senses offered by physician Henrik Wulff, who has made significant contributions to our thinking in philosophy of medicine. These senses of causal relation include necessary, sufficient, and contributory (Wulff 1981, 56–57), which are well recognized in contemporary medical literature on the nature of rational diagnosis and treatment (also see Gøtzsche 2007, 52–56).

To begin with, "[f]actor X is a *necessary* determinant, if X always precedes Y, which of course does not imply that Y always succeeds X" (Wulff 1981, 56). It can be illustrated as follows (Gøtzsche 2007, 54):

$$\nearrow$$
$$X \rightarrow Y$$
$$\searrow$$

Figure 2.1 Necessary causal relation.

An example here is the relationship between a determinant cause "tubercle bacilli" and an effect "pulmonary tuberculosis." In this case, the disease pulmonary tuberculosis (Y) is always preceded by the introduction of the tubercle bacilli (X), but the introduction of the tubercle bacilli does not always lead to the disease pulmonary tuberculosis. One can be exposed to the bacilli and not express pulmonary tuberculosis. In the case of a gender-specific disease, the gender-specific determinant (X) will be a necessary condition of the disease (Y) if the disease (Y) is always preceded by the gender-specific determinant (X). The clinical condition called fragile X is an example here. Fragile X is a genetic condition that involves the expansion of a single trinucleotide gene sequence CGG on the X chromosome (National Fragile X Foundation 2011). Given this, some will prefer to call it a sex-linked disease. Fragile X results in a host of physical, intellectual, emotional, and behavioral features in primarily males. Fragile X is always preceded by the introduction of genetic traits, but the introduction of the genetic traits does not always lead to the disease. One can have the sex-linked traits and yet not express the disease in cases when the expansion of the single trinucleotide gene sequence CGG is not sufficient to express the disease (although one could say that the patient is presymptomatic for the condition).

A second sense of "cause" is referred to as "sufficient." "Factor X is a *sufficient* determinant, if X always leads to Y," which "does not imply that Y is always preceded by X" (Wulff 1981, 57). This can be illustrated as follows (Gøtzsche 2007, 54):

$$\searrow$$
$$X \rightarrow Y$$
$$\nearrow$$

Figure 2.2 Sufficient causal relation.

An example here is the relationship between the causal determinant "lack of iron in the food" (X) and the effect "anemia" (Y). If the body is not properly supplied with iron over a period of time, then anemia is always the result. But anemia frequently has different causes, such as problems with red blood cells and their ability to carry iron in the body. In the case of gender-specific disease, the gender-specific determinant (X) always leads to the disease (Y), but there are other determinants or paths by which the disease can occur. Color blindness is an example here (Color Blindness 2011). Color blindness involves a decreased ability to perceive differences between colors and can be caused by genetic determinants on the X chromosome. When it does, it affects males more than females. Yet, there are other ways to develop color blindness. For instance, a variety of neurological, optical, or chemical determinants can bring about color blindness.

A third sense of "cause" is referred to as "contributory." In medicine, "[s]ome determinants are neither necessary nor sufficient, but only *contributory*. This term is used if some factor X leads to an increased probability of Y, though X does not lead to Y and Y is not always preceded by X" (Wulff 1981, 57). This can be illustrated as follows (Gøtzsche 2007, 54):

$$X \to Y$$

Figure 2.3 Contributory causal relation.

An example here is arterial hypertension: "Arterial hypertension, for instance, is a contributory determinant of myocardial infarction as myocardial infarction is more frequent among hypertensives than among others, and that probably means that some patients with a myocardial infarction would not have developed the disease if they had not had hypertension" (Gøtzsche 2007, 55). In the case of gender-specific disease, some gender-specific factors (X) lead to an increased probability of disease (Y), though the factors (X) do not lead directly to the disease (Y) and the disease (Y) is not always preceded by the factors (X). Consider systemic lupus erythematosus, a condition that primarily affects women. Lupus is a chronic inflammatory disease in which an individual's immune system attacks healthy tissues and organs. Studies show that genetic variants contribute to an increased probability of lupus, although at this time it is unclear how the genetic variants lead to lupus and lupus is not always preceded by these genetic variants. Stress (a general category of determinants), hormones, smoking, and certain infections also play a role in the expression of lupus (Warner 2011).

As presented here, a naturalist view of disease causation finds great support in gender-specific medicine. It assists in identifying conditions that are necessary to produce effects, ones that are sufficient to produce effects, or ones that contribute to the likelihood of an effect's occurring. This approach to understanding gender-specific disease is in keeping with an influential assumption in medicine that gender and disease are real entities that can be known through reliable empirical methodologies and causal models of the relation between gender and disease can be generated. In medicine, where the data are always statistical, causal factors will usually be identified as contributory with the hope that medicine will be able to move toward a more rigorous sense of causal contribution and the development of more specifically designed therapies for a particular disease. This is the hope for gender-specific medicine as well (Institute of Medicine 2001a; Legato 2004a, 2010b).

CREATING GENDER-SPECIFIC DISEASE

A naturalist account of gender-specific disease is attractive because it fits within a prevailing view in medicine that gender, disease, and their relation can be studied using the tools of science. But it is not without its limits.

Nominalist View of Gender and Sex

Despite the attractiveness of a naturalist's account of gender, a naturalist view of gender as a real or objective "fact" that is expressed in two kinds may be misleading. As much as we may wish to reduce gender to a "fact" about the social construction of sex that comes in two kinds, gender defies this classification and description. As Chapter 1 reviewed, gender refers to a myriad of expressions. Sometimes in medicine it refers to "the social construction of sex," whatever that might mean to the spokesperson and/ or listener. Sometimes it refers to a psychological phenomenon, for which a host of terminology has been developed to talk about its distinct aspects, such as "gender identity," "gender roles," and "sexual orientation," all of which turn on interpretations particular to certain individuals and cultures. Here gender identity "refers to a person's self-representation as male or female (with the caveat that some individuals may not identify exclusively with either)" (Hughes et al. 2006, 554). Gender role "describes the psychological characteristics that are sexually dimorphic within the general population, such as toy preferences and physical aggression" (Hughes et al. 2006, 554). Sexual orientation "refers to the direction(s) of erotic interest (heterosexual, bisexual, homosexual) and includes behaviours, fantasies, and attractions" (Hughes et al. 2006, 554). Other times gender refers to a set of social power relationships. Gender serves to draw attention to how social systems support and maintain gender performance roles and to the problem of stereotyping members of certain genders. Other times, gender refers to a continuum, as opposed to a phenomenon expressed in two kinds: "An individual may display characteristics more typical of the opposite sex, and a person's sense of gender may change over the course of a life time" (Institute of Medicine 2001a, 17). In short, an analysis of gender appears to involve more than bench science "facts" about an individual; it involves individualized and particular interpretations that bring together a host of psychological, social, and subjective considerations. A *nominalist view of gender* begins to emerge.

Part of the difficulty in establishing a naturalist view of gender is rooted in the difficulty of establishing a naturalist view of sex. In the last century, biologists and clinicians have recognized that human beings display a range of sexual diversity (Reis 2007). Despite controversies surrounding the nomenclature, standard clinical texts still report that there are those who fall in so-called exclusive genetic classes (e.g., a normal homologous XX [female] or non-homologous XY [male]). There are those who do not fall within either class (e.g., those with Turner's syndrome involving XO or a single X chromosome, and those with Klinefelter's syndrome involving the presence of one or two additional X chromosomes in a male). There are those who fall in both: a so-called "true hermaphrodite" possesses at least one ovary and at least one testis, or at least one ovotestis, a "male pseudo-hermaphrodite" has testes (and not ovaries or ovotestes) and an XY chromosomal complement, and a "female pseudohermaphrodite" has ovaries (and not testes or ovotestes) and an XX chromosomal complement (Dreger et al. 2005, 729).

In the 1990s, Brown University biologist Anne Fausto-Sterling became notable for arguing in favor of five sexes: "Biologically speaking, there are many gradations running from female to male; and depending on how one calls the shots, one can argue that along the spectrum lie at least five sexes—and perhaps even more" (Fausto-Sterling 1993, 21). She includes the three variations of hermaphrodite as additional sexual categories (she refers to them as "intersexual"), but recognizes that human sexuality is more of a continuum than a dimorphism. In her later work, Fausto-Sterling revises her five-sex theory and argues that it would be better to move away from basing an account of sex on genitals, which is the basis for the nomenclature of hermaphroditism, which is fraught with problems. Instead, one should adopt the language of intersexuality and acknowledge that "people come in a wider assortment of identities and characteristics than mere genitals can distinguish" (Fausto-Sterling 2000a, 22; 2005). Studies show that at least 1.7% of the human population expresses sexual diversity or are intersexual (Fausto-Sterling 2000b). Some say the prevalence is about .018% (Sax 2002) and others say that one in 1,500 to one in 2,000 of live births exhibit some degree of sexual ambiguity (Intersex Society of North America 2011 [2008]; Dreger 2004, 139). Regardless of the differences, there is emerging agreement that the concept of intersexuality leads us to rethink our understanding of sex in terms of specified gonadal tissues.

Further, to arrive at an account of intersexuality, one will first have to get participants to agree on what counts as intersex or intersexual—which involves agreeing on what counts as "male" and as "female." Such is difficult to do. As philosopher of science and medical humanities Alice Dreger (1998, 2004) has raised, most judgments about intersexuality are made by the bedside and involve observing a patient. How small does a penis have to be before the organism counts as intersexual? How large does a clitoris have to be? What kinds of sexual practices are typically engaged in by "females," "males," and the "intersexes"? When sex chromosomal data are gathered, does one count sex chromosomal anomalies as intersexual if there is no apparent external sexual ambiguity? How does one account for those who are born without external expressions of intersexuality, but who have genetic factors associated with such a diagnosis? What is the test for intersexuality—penis size, clitoris size, testicular or ovarian tissue, hormone levels, etc.? Dreger states the problem with clarity: "One quickly runs into a problem . . . when trying to define 'key' or 'essential' feminine and masculine anatomy. In fact, any close study of sexual anatomy results in a loss of faith that there is a simple, "natural" sex distinction that will not break down in the face of certain anatomical, behavioral, or philosophical challenges" (Dreger 2004, 139). In the end, then, we arrive at a *nominalist view of sex* and the view that there is no "natural" human sexuality that we can know outside the boundaries of our assumptions, claims, and expectations (also see Lorber and Moore 2002; Hubbard 2004, 65).

Nominalist View of Disease

Similarly, a naturalist view of disease may be misleading. Disease may not be discovered in nature as naturalists think it can be. The late-eighteenth-century pathologist Xavier Bichat (1771–1802) criticized the seventeenth-century clinicians for thinking that the diseases they referred to were discoverable natural entities. For Bichat, the "ancient practitioners" William Cullen (1710–1790) and F.B. Sauvages (1701–1767), "erred in their classifications" (Bichat 1981 [1801], 168) because they confined themselves "to the simple observation of symptoms" (Bichat 1981 [1801], 167) along the lines of Sydenham's suggestions. These practitioners wrongly considered certain sets of symptoms, such as *critici* or fever, and *dolorosi* or painful disease, as "essential" maladies. Early-nineteenth-century physician F.J.V. Broussais (1772–1838) (1981 [1821]) similarly voiced concerns about filling "the nosological [clinical classificatory] framework with groups of most arbitrarily formed symptoms . . . which do not represent the affections of different organs, that is, the real disease" (Broussais 1981 [1821], Vol. 2, 646). Although Bichat and Broussais held that the real essence of disease was to be found elsewhere and specifically in the etiological properties of disease, they are relevant here insofar as they warned clinicians against thinking that they had discovered the real or "ontological" essence of disease when they did not.

Notably, in the twentieth century, psychiatrist Thomas Szasz (1961) has supported a *nominalist view of disease*. Although Szasz does support a naturalist view of somatic disease, he is a nominalist about mental disease. Szasz argues that mental disease cannot exist because it is not a result of tissue damage or tissue dysfunction. "The concept of illness, whether bodily or mental, implies deviation from some clearly defined norm. In the case of physical illness, the norm is the structural and functional integrity of the human body" (Szasz 1991 [1970], 23). After questioning the norm of mental illness, Szasz provocatively claims that mental illness is a "myth." When he says that mental illness is a myth, he does not mean that there are no mental conditions, such as sadness and anxiety, which debilitate individuals and lead to pain and suffering. He is rather interested in showing how mental disease has been used for all sorts of socio-political purposes from labeling patients to incarcerating social deviants: "The ideology of insanity . . . has succeeded in depriving vast numbers of people . . . of a vocabulary of their own in which to frame their predicament without paying homage to a psychiatric perspective that diminishes man as a person and oppresses him as a citizen" (Szasz 1991 [1970], 5). Szasz calls for the relinquishment of the notion of mental disease and for increased work on the biological basis of mental illness for purposes of grounding psychiatry in somatic medicine.

Szasz's critique of mental disease classifications has become a rallying call for those who draw attention to the medicalization of illness, dysfunction, and disorders. Medical sociologist Peter Conrad (2007) defines medicalization as "a process by which nonmedical problems become defined and treated as medical problems" (4). In this process, non-medical problems are "defined in medical terms, described using medical language, understood through the adoption of a medical framework, or 'treated' with a medical intervention" (Conrad 2007, 5). In a lengthy analysis, Conrad illustrates how, over the past half-century, the social terrain of health and illness has been transformed. What were once considered normal human events and common human problems, such as birth, menstruation, pregnancy, menopause, alcoholism, obesity, and aging, are transformed into medical conditions. Conrad warns that the medicalization of illness, dysfunctions, and disorders have far-reaching implications in our lives. It places labels on clinical events that might better be understood as part of "normal" life and instructs that such "normal" events should be treated with medical interventions.

The medicalization or construction of disease is a complex matter. "Construction" may mean many things to many people. Philosopher of science Ian Hacking has examined a wide range of books and articles with titles of the form "the social construction of X" or "constructing X." He argues that when something is said to be "constructed," this is shorthand for at least the following two claims:

(1) In the present state of affairs, X is taken for granted (1999, 12).
(2) X need not have existed, or need not be at all as it is. X, or X as it is at present, is not determined by the nature of things; it is not inevitable (1999, 6).

Hacking adds that the following claims are also often, though not always, implied by the use of the phrase "construction":

(3) X is quite bad as it is.

(4) We would be much better off if X were done away with, or at least radically transformed (1999, 6).

Applied to our discussion of disease, the claim that disease is constructed can mean that the clinical event, as currently understood, is taken for granted or is not an inevitable result of biology. We assume that the clinical event is a disease because we have no reason to challenge this assumption or we assume that the clinical event is determined by biological processes. In addition, it can mean that our view of a clinical event is harmful, and should be modified or eliminated. We label a clinical event as disease because we deem the event as harmful to a patient, group of patients, or society, and therefore should be done away with or changed. (This point is developed further in the next chapter.) These varying interpretations illustrate how humans create disease.

Nominalist View of Disease Causation

On a nominalist view, gender-specific disease results establish an association between "gender-specific factors" and "disease." For some, this type of association is a form of "causal constructivism." British philosopher David Hume (1711–1776) (1978 [1739–40]) provides a classic account of causal constructivism. Granted, this does not appear to be a popular view found among clinical practitioners and researchers today, but bear with me as I show its relevancy in gender-specific medical discussions. Hume argues that causal connection is nothing more than constantly conjoined events, when two events are in "succession" and have "contiguity" (1978 [1739–40], 76): "I find . . . that whatever objects are consider'd as causes of effects, are contiguous; and that nothing can operate in a time or place, which is ever so little remov'd from those of its existence" (Hume 1978 [1739–40], 75). According to Hume, assignments of causal connection are based on our experiences of events as sequential and in turn expected to occur; nothing more essential or substantial can be known about the events. In the case of gender-specific disease, the determination of the causal connection between gender-specific factors and disease is a reflection of what we single out as efficacious in bringing about disease. Here efficacious will be a function of what appears to be constant and conjoined in our experience. In this way, our understanding of causal connection tells us more about how the human mind works than about the essential structure of nature.

Philosopher of science Paul Thagard (who defends a naturalist and not a nominalist account of disease causation) helps us understand how a *nominalist view of disease causation* has come to find support in medicine. According to Thagard, in order to determine the cause of disease, the clinician-scientist must be clear about what disease is being explained (1999, 129). This is not an easy task because all accounts of disease are limited and must contend with a lack of evidence (Thagard 1999, 131). It took four hundred years to understand scurvy and tuberculosis because of the difficulty in assessing the multiplicity of possible causes and background assumptions in our views. Gender-specific practitioners face similar challenges in establishing what gender-specific factors bring about what kinds of disease.

Further, in order to determine the cause(s) of disease, the clinician-scientist must clarify the relevant cause(s) of a disease. This is not an easy task, given that biological and environmental factors dually contribute to disease expression (Thagard 1999, 130). The inference that a factor is a cause of a disease is based on explanatory coherence. We can infer that the factor causes the disease if this hypothesis is part of the best explanation given a full range of evidence. But, according to Thagard, determining "that the factor and the disease are positively correlated (i.e., that the probability of the disease given the factor is greater than the probability of disease without the factor) does not suffice to show that the factor causes the disease" (Thagard 1999, 129). The correlation might be spurious, or accidental. This can be illustrated as follows (Gøtzsche 2007, 55).

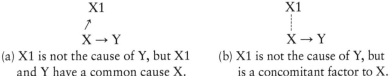

(a) X1 is not the cause of Y, but X1 and Y have a common cause X.   (b) X1 is not the cause of Y, but is a concomitant factor to X.

Figure 2.4a–b Spurious causal relation.

As seen in Figure 2.4, even if the correlation between causal factors (X1) and disease (Y) appears genuine, it may not indicate a causal relation if X1 and Y have a common cause (X) or if X1 is a concomitant factor to X in causing Y. In the case of Figure 2.4 above, consider a case in which a population has been vaccinated before it was hit by an epidemic. Let's say that the vaccinated individuals were infected less frequently than the non-vaccinated ones. A tempting conclusion is to say that the vaccination was effective and contributed to the prevention of infection. Our consideration of spurious causal relations reminds us that there may be other possible explanations. Perhaps those who were vaccinated were less vulnerable to the infection at the start. Perhaps those who were vaccinated practiced a certain lifestyle that protected them against the infection or were less vulnerable to the infection because of some physiological reason. Then, the relationship between the vaccination and protection against the infection may be due to a common cause (called a *confounder*) (Figure 2.4a). It is also possible that the vaccination was a *concomitant* factor to the real determining factor (Figure 2.4b). Say that those who were vaccinated were told to also practice a particular hygienic practice (e.g., boiling their water) and that this precaution protected them against the infectious disease. The point is that in the case of gender-specific diseases, researchers and clinicians will need to rule out confounding and concomitant etiological factors when determining what gender-specific factors cause certain disease conditions.

Further, according to Thagard, there can also be "causal beliefs" (1999, 130), that is, taken-for-granted associations between so-called causal factors and diseases that are not questioned. Beliefs in medicine are not always bad, for they can provide impetus to pursue hunches in research. There are numerous hunches about what constitutes a gender-specific disease that are based on day-to-day observations of what diseases affect women in unique ways. But left unquestioned, they can be problematic in medical inquiry. Here one is reminded of the causal beliefs undergirding Aristotle's view that the female was "a sort of natural deficiency" (Aristotle 1984, 726.b.33) and Dr. Dirix's view that all diseases of women were rooted in the uterus so that all women's disease were a "disease of the womb" (quoted in Smith-Rosenberg and Rosenberg 1981, 284) (see Chapter 1). More recently, we have become well aware of the claims made in the early years of the AIDS epidemic about the causal relation between being gay and having AIDS (Treichler 1999).

The bottom line is that there are numerous reasons to hold that an etiological account of gender-specific disease represents a name that is created as opposed to an ontological reality. The difficulty we have in defining disease and determining its relevant causes highlights the vulnerability of developing definitive naturalist accounts of gender-specific disease. Further, given that data in medicine is statistical, it is not difficult to see that our causal accounts heavily rely on claims about how events are sequentially organized and such sequential organization may be more of a reflection of the ideas in our mind than of the essential structure of clinical reality.

DISCOVERING A CREATION

Despite the attractiveness of a nominalist view of gender-specific disease, there *is* something we can say about gender and sex differences in disease expression and treatment. Anything does not go in our understanding of gender-specific disease. There are limited expressions of gender (e.g., women, men, girls, boys, gay, lesbian, transgender, etc.) as well as genetic sexuality (e.g., XX and XY, intersex, etc.), gonadal sexuality (e.g., ovaries, testes), hormonal sexuality (e.g., specified levels of estrogens and androgens), and genital sexuality (e.g., clitoris, penis). There are limited expressions of disease, or of biological dysfunction and complaints patients bring to the clinic. There are limited expressions of the ways in which we understand disease causation. Limited expressions of gender, sex, and dysfunction are a function of the designs of nature (where nature is the term we give for what we "find" or "discover" in the world in which we inhabit) *and* the labels clinicians, patients, and others use to classify and explain such phenomena. These limitations and expressions of gender, sexuality, and disease are supported by what clinicians and others observe, the language they use, and the choices humans make.

As Thagard contends, a simple nominalist view of disease and disease etiology is unable to explain developments in medicine and science (Thagard 1999, 239). It is incapable of explaining many aspects of scientific practice, such as the recalcitrance of experimentation, the reliability of instruments, the causal efficacy of theory, and the realist nature of scientific discourse. In other words, medicine has been successful in delivering accounts of disease that fit with prevailing experimental data, are measurable around the world, work in clinical practice, and form the basis of an international dialogue among clinicians, scientists, and patients. Although they certainly do not know everything about disease, medical practitioners and scientists have indeed been able to agree on matters concerning disease and have been able to treat patients successfully.

It seems, then, that both naturalists and nominalists have something to offer in thinking about the character of gender-specific disease. Consider a "both/and" perspective when it comes to navigating between naturalist and nominalist accounts of gender-specific disease. Here I will begin with an example provided by philosopher Ian Hacking. Replacing "quarks" with "gender-specific disease," consider the claim that "gender-specific disease is constructed." On one reading, this means that gender-specific disease itself is not "inevitable" or "determined by the nature of things." It is rather a creation of the mind and the conventions we use. On another reading, the claim that "gender-specific disease is constructed" can mean that our *idea* (or conceptualization, or understanding) of gender-specific disease is not "inevitable" or "determined by the nature of things." Hacking argues that, if the second reading is taken, there need not always be a conflict between saying that a "quark," or in our case "gender-specific disease," is "constructed" and saying that it is "real" (Hacking 1999, 29–30). This is the case because there is no denial of reality, but rather an admission that the ideas, concepts, labels, and names that make up our concept are constructed. When it comes to gender-specific disease, then, we can say that that gender-specific disease is discovered as well as created.

This view supports what I call a *methodological naturalist view of gender-specific disease.* A methodological naturalist view of gender-specific disease supports the view that investigation of gender-specific disease and natural phenomena provides information about a clinical world that we do not simply make up. It supports the view that empirical investigation into natural phenomena provides reliable information about the order and structure of natural phenomena. Yet, it leaves room for the recognition that human knowers in part create clinical reality. They create the particular language used to talk about clinical reality and the goals that are sought to be achieved.

A methodological naturalist view of gender-specific disease is not a *metaphysical* naturalist view (Ruse 2005). It does not claim access to the ultimate structure of reality. It makes no claim that the natural world is metaphysically or essentially this or that. It makes no such claim because it cannot. It does not take a stand on the ultimate structure of reality because it recognizes that it is constrained by the methodology that it employs to advance knowledge claims. In the case of medicine, the methodology that is employed is an empirical one, which is unable to make any claims about ultimate or absolute questions. A methodological naturalist view recognizes that we do not completely make up our world, that empirical methods do provide knowledge of the world, and that there are limits with the knowledge claims that are made.

SUMMARY

A *methodological naturalist account of gender-specific disease* recognizes that gender, disease, and their relation are discovered as well as created. Gender-specific disease describes gender-specific biological dysfunction via etiological laws, generalizations, or associations. It singles out gender-specific phenomena in biological functioning and interprets it according to current methodological standards. In this description, gender is neither simply a biological nor social construction, disease is neither simply an entity out there to be discovered nor simply a construction, and the relation between gender and disease is neither simply determined by a single causal variable nor is completely fabricated. Although gender-specific disease is "real" in the sense in which it is a manifestation of "nature," it is interpreted within our frames of references. Gender-specific disease is "both/and" discovered and created.

3 Gender-Specific Disease
Prescriptive Analysis

PRESCRIBING CLINICAL PHENOMENA

This chapter explores how gender-specific disease provides a prescriptive account of human biological dysfunction that differs between the genders. The chapter employs the language of gender and sex found in gender-specific disease and submits it to further analysis in order to illustrate the evaluative dimensions of the concepts. Using the language found in the philosophy of medicine literature, and adopting it to discussions about gender-specific disease, it contrasts a *neutralist* with a *normative* account of gender-specific disease. Here the term "neutralist" comes from the Latin *neuter*, which means "neither" or "neither one or the other." The term "normative" comes from the Latin *norma*, which means "rule" or "principle." Whereas a neutralist account of gender-specific disease holds that the concept of gender-specific disease is value-neutral, a normative account holds that it is value-ladened. The chapter argues in favor of a *normativist view of gender-specific disease*, and one that recognizes that the values that inform disease are not simply subjective. A normative account of gender-specific disease recognizes that gender-specific disease serves to judge a clinical phenomenon as dysfunctional, to enlist the actions of health care professionals, and to guide treatment recommendations.

THE FACT OF GENDER-SPECIFIC DISEASE

The great success of medicine in contemporary culture is said to be due largely to medicine's adoption of an objective empirical methodology that provides reliable and useful data and assessments. Logical positivists of the early twentieth century were particularly instrumental in supporting these efforts in science and medicine. Logical positivism is a name given by A.E. Blumberg and Herbert Feigl in 1931 to a set of philosophical discussions put forward by the Vienna Circle, academics who set out to produce a scientifically based philosophy, to eliminate all transcendental metaphysics, including values, and to emphasize the importance of mathematics and theoretical physics. Although the Vienna Circle dissolved in the early 1930s, its ideas spread to England and the U.S. (Pojman 2003, 465–66).

Its influence remains today in contemporary medicine and science, and in major areas of philosophy.

The Vienna Circle's influence is particularly evident in how we understand the nature of, and relation between, facts and values. Here "fact" is understood as a claim about the world which is empirically confirmable or falsifiable. Such a claim "either describes or asserts the existence of some event or object. Its objective is presumably to say what is true, and factual statements are thus either true or false" (Beauchamp 1982, 349). This is in contrast to a "value," which is taken to be "an evaluative statement or judgment concerning what is, for example, good, right, or virtuous" (Beauchamp 1982, 349). A value expresses what *ought* to be the case, as opposed to what *is* the case. For logical positivists, anyone who tries to move in an argument from purely factual premises (so-called "is" statements) to evaluative conclusions (so-called "ought" statements) errs. This is because factual statements do not entail evaluative ones. In other words, one cannot derive an "ought" from an "is." The gap between facts and values, the "is" and "ought," has come to be known as the entailment gap, and the attempt to derive value statements from factual ones is known as the "naturalistic fallacy" (Beauchamp 1982, 245, 351).

Value-Neutral View of Gender and Sex

In the case of medicine, a value-neutral account of gender-specific disease is attractive for many of the reasons that have already been considered in discussions of a naturalist account of gender-specific disease presented in Chapter 2. A value-neutral account of gender-specific disease fits with a prevailing view in medicine that disease nosologies and nosographies are, and should be, void of motives, bias, and socio-political motives. Recall Dr. Miller's critique (2005) of Dr. Legato's use of "gender" as opposed to "sex" in the title of her edited volumes on gender-specific medicine. Miller's encouragement to clinicians to replace "gender" with "sex" in their discussions of gender-specific disease is in keeping with the Vienna Circle's call to jettison non-empirical (and thus non-verifiable) language and ideas from medical scientific discourse.

At first blush, it may be challenging to conceive of gender as value-neutral. Part of this has to do with the term itself, which has come to be defined in a number of ways, and most widely as the social construction of sex. In that it is conceived as a social construction of sex, gender is open to the interpretations and values of a given society. Nevertheless, there are those (e.g., the Institute of Medicine 2001a) who attempt a value-neutral account of gender. As discussed in the previous chapter, this value-free component is sex, and sex is seen to be the biological basis or fact underlying gender. In its report, *Exploring the Biological Contributions to Human Health: Does Sex Matter?* (2001a), the Institute of Medicine forwards a *neutralist sense of gender and sex*. As we have learned in the previous chapter, it defines gender as "[a] person's self-representation as male or female, or how that person is responded to by social institutions based on the individual's gender presentation" (Institute of Medicine 2001a, 17). Whereas the Institute of Medicine does not discuss the role of values in disease nosology and nosography, it seeks to define gender in terms of its biological roots. As it says, "[g]ender is rooted in biology and shaped by environment and experience" (2001a, 17). The Institute of Medicine further states that "gender is a continuum. An individual may display characteristics more typical of the opposite sex, and a person's sense of gender may change over the course of a life-time" (2001a, 17). Here gender is again explained in terms of sex, which is understood to be "dimorphic." As the Institute of Medicine says, "[w]ith some exceptions, individuals are either chromosomally XX and developmentally female or chromosomally XY and developmentally male" (2001a, 17). In that gender is rooted in biology or sex, and can be explained in terms of a deviation from it, it entails an important value-free component, one that can be the focus of scientific study in gender-specific medicine.

In addition, given that gender is seen to be rooted in biology, the Institute of Medicine gives precedence to physiology over the more value-infused disciplines of sociology and psychology, and gender becomes a legitimate focus of (value-free) bioscientific research. It recognizes the need "to look at sex and gender as part of a single system in which social elements act with biological elements to produce the body" (2001a, 19). It holds that scientific ground will be broken when the "biological questions . . . are posed as a result of an approach that examines how factors outside the body are translated into differences between male and female bodies" (2001a, 19). In reducing sociological and psychological research to biomedical research, the Institute of Medicine suggests that a certain area of research (i.e., the biomedical) is more important than others (e.g., the sociological, psychological), thus supporting the view that a value-neutral approach to gender-specific disease is preferred.

Value-Neutral View of Disease

The need for a value-free way to talk about clinical reality also emerges in discussions about disease. Physician Thomas Sydenham sought to remove all speculative thought from discussions of clinical classifications and descriptions. Whereas Sydenham did not discuss the role of values in disease nosology and nosography, one can see him playing a role in encouraging the development of a *neutralist account of disease* and the removal of evaluative claims from clinical discourse. In the preface to the third edition of his 1676 *Observationes medicae*, Sydenham said: "In writing the history of a disease, every philosophical hypothesis whatsoever, that has previously occupied the mind of the author, should lie in abeyance" (1981 [1676], 147). For Sydenham, a clinician's history of disease was infected with speculative thinking that distracted attention from cataloguing the empirical conditions of disease for purposes of developing reliable diagnoses. Sydenham petitioned clinicians to observe and document the "natural phenomena of the disease" (147). Here "natural" refers to that which is separate and distinct from the observer and is given to us. For him, "[t]rue medicine consists in the discovery of the real indication" (155) of the disease, unfiltered through distracting speculative lenses.

More recently, philosopher Christopher Boorse has been a consistent and vocal supporter of a neutralist view of disease. According to Boorse, the function of a physiological process is determined by its contributions to physiological goals (1997, 21). A "function" is "a causal contribution to a goal" (Boorse 1997, 8–9) and the goal may "involve individual survival, survival of the genes, equilibrium, etc." (Boorse 1997, 9). Here Boorse relies on philosopher G. Sommerhoff's (1950, 6) account of goal-directedness, namely, tendencies that are directed toward the fulfillment of specific and mutually interrelated ends. For Boorse, this sense of goal-directedness is value-neutral. Disease involves a deficiency of the natural functional organization of the organism. By "deficiency" of function, Boorse means "simply less function, less contribution to the goals, than average" (Boorse 1997, 21). For him, deficiency of function "is an arithmetic, not evaluative, concept" (1997, 21). To interfere with or disrupt a functional process is to lower its degree of achievement of physiological goals and this can be descriptively defined. In the end, disease is a value-neutral concept.

Value-Neutral View of Disease Causation

With regard to determining the relation between gender-specific variables and disease, there is a long-standing assumption in medicine that *statements of causal relation are value-neutral*. As the discussion in the last chapter illustrates, in determining a cause, clinicians move from the descriptive to the experimental and establish the (value-free) conditions that must be in place to facilitate the scientific study of the origins and mechanisms of a disease. They seek to provide accounts of determinant conditions that are necessary to produce gender-specific disease, ones that are sufficient to produce gender-specific disease, and ones that contribute to the likelihood of occurrence of a gender-specific disease (Institute of Medicine 2001a). These accounts of causal relation rely on formal and informal statistical methods to determine what causes bring about certain effects. Such statistical methods rely on math, and math is seen to be value-neutral with regard to possible ends, actions, and cognitive objects (Sundström 1998).

Recall Boorse's account of disease reviewed in the last chapter. According to Boorse, disease is biological dysfunction that is statistically abnormal. It is a dysfunction in that it is a failure of some internal mechanism to perform a natural function, and natural function is understood in explanatory terms as an effect that plays a role in shaping the biological mechanism that causes it. It is statistical abnormality in that it is mathematically calculated to be an internal state that depresses a functional ability below species-typical levels. In that disease is biological dysfunction which is statistically abnormal, Boorse contends that this view of disease causation is value-free (Boorse 1975, 1977).

THE VALUE OF GENDER-SPECIFIC DISEASE

A closer look at the concept of gender-specific disease indicates that the ideal of its value-neutrality may be unattainable. Recall that the prior chapter concluded that the concept of gender-specific disease is in part discovered and in part created. Because gender-specific disease is in part created, it is a function of choices we as knowers make about how to assemble the observations, data, and evidence that are gathered in the world in light of our ends and goals. Here choice involves values. Knowers select among options for purposes of achieving certain ends as opposed to others.

Normative View of Gender and Sex

To be more specific, *gender* serves a normative role in medicine. As has already been recognized, gender typically refers to the social construction of sex. In this way, gender supports judgments or norms about how individuals ought to be, act, and so forth. As Legato herself recognizes, "gender is the phenotype that comes out of embedding a male or female in his or her culture. Societies *award* different resources to men and women, assign them different roles, and *value* them differently" (Legato 2004b, xv). On one prominent model, for example, to be "good" at being female or feminine, one should be nurturing, emotional, cooperative, sexually restrained, pretty, etc.; to be good at being a male or masculine, one should be strong, active, independent, rational, sexually aggressive, handsome, etc. (Achterberg 1991, Part IV). In such cases, the achievement of such norms are typically rewarded. This is the message advanced by health care professionals who prescribe hormone therapies (Wilson 1966; Spake 2002; Houck 2006) and cosmetic surgeons who promote the benefits of facial lifts and alterations (American Society of Plastic Surgeons Overall Trends 2008). Alternatively, the lack of achievement of such norms typically meets with negative evaluation. As the history of medicine illustrates, if a woman's behavior violated expected gender-role norms, her behavior was attributed to various physical or mental illnesses and in turn treated in a variety of ways—with labels such as "hysterical" (Acocella 1998), with pharmaceutical agents such as antidepressants (Greenspan 1993; Weissman and Olfson 1995; Hirschbein 2006), and with gynecological surgeries such as hysterectomies and clitorectomies (Waisberg and Paige 1988; Broverman et al. 1970).

The normative role of gender extends beyond evaluation of praiseworthiness and blameworthiness. Gender serves to draw attention to how social systems support and maintain gender performance roles and to the problem of stereotyping members of certain genders. As feminist philosopher Drucilla Cornell (2004) points out, "gender as an analytic category was the creation of second-wave feminism" (Cornell 2004, 37), where second-wave feminism refers to a movement beginning in the 1960s in the U.S. that called for equality between women and men. The term gender "was used to expose a lacunae in literary, social, political, and scientific work, and to show that any history told without gender missed the crucial developments and struggles various literary texts, social movements, political institutions, and scientific discoveries were trying to elaborate" (Cornell 2004, 37). More specifically, it was developed to openly dispute "the idea that biological difference between the sexes should ever be used—even affirmatively—to justify women's participation as citizens" (Cornell 2004, 37). One might think here of the efforts taken by members of the women's health movement to criticize the lack of inclusion of women in clinical research projects because of their child-bearing roles (Moncher and Douglas 2004).

Further, the term "gender" is used to highlight "that 'woman' does not denote a common identity and, even more radically, that it is ethically and politically undesirable for feminism to seek in the category of woman a universal basis for its ethics and politics" (Cornell 2004, 39). The thinking here is that when the concept of woman is universalized, it privileges hegemonic Western imperialistic ideas concerning gender, male superiority, and women's oppression. Drawing on feminist philosopher Judith Butler (1990), Cornell claims that a universal or essentialist view of woman adopts "the moral injunction of heterosexual normativity that has been integral to our very conceptualization of women" (Cornell 2004, 40). It assumes all women are the same and that all women are similarly related to men. As Butler says, "[i]f one 'is' a woman, that is surely not all one is; the term fails to be exhaustive . . . because gender is not always constituted coherently or consistently in different historical contexts" (Butler 1990, 3). Butler's crucial insight, according to Cornell (2004, 40), is that gender is not a set of fixed traits but rather serves as a form of repetition of imposed norms that decide not only how our bodies come to matter, but how they are given meaning. As much as science and medicine may want to reduce "woman" and "female" to a simple biological phenomenon, it will not be able to do so.

Along with gender, *sex serves a normative role* in medicine. As much as the Institute of Medicine (2001a, 175–76) may wish us to distinguish the meaning and use of the terms "sex" and "gender," this hard and fast distinction between a "fact" and a "value" may not accurately reflect reality. As is well recognized today, nature (e.g., sex) and nurture (e.g., gender) are not so separate and distinct. Genetic science provides extensive data to illustrate that nature and nurture operate together, albeit in different ways, nature at times contributing more (as in the case of a "single-gene" disease) and nurture at times contributing more (as in the case of an environmentally-induced disease). But, as far as humans can know, nature is never without nurture, and nurture never without nature. Humans are embodied beings living in environments and environments are constituted by expressions in nature. Given this, it becomes increasingly difficult to define sex as a "fact" that is separate and distinct from gender. Sex draws attention to how we evaluate chromosomal identity, reproductive fitness, hormonal functioning, and organ structure. It reflects how medical and social systems support and maintain sexual performance roles. It, along with gender, is both nature and nurture.

Borrowing from philosopher of science and medical humanities Alice Dreger (1998, 2004), to arrive at an account of sex, one will first have to get experts to agree on what counts as sex. There will be questions concerning how sex is verified, and what calculations go into determining when one is considered a member of one sex over another. As Dreger reminds us, such calculations are typically not based on detailed scientific assessment. They are based on observations by the bed- or chair-side and on reports patients provide. A determination of sex is typically based not on sophisticated genetic analysis of the sex chromosomes, but rather observations that occur upon birth or in the physician's office and reports that are gathered in the clinic. Such observations and reports do not occur in a vacuum. They are influenced by how medicine evaluates normality and what our medical and social systems support and maintain.

For Dreger, the creation of a "natural" sex distinction turns on evaluative assumptions about what is normal. As she says, "[t]he strict conception of 'normal' sexual anatomy and 'normal' sex behavior that underlies prevailing treatment protocols is arguably sexist in its asymmetrical treatment of reproductive potential and definitions of anatomical 'adequacy'" (2004, 143). For Dreger, decisions regarding sex and gender assignments are inseparable from a heterosexual matrix, which has a longstanding history and is assumed to be settled. Even within heterosexuality, a rich array of sexual practices is reduced to vaginal penetration of sexual features to a clitoris or penis of a certain length (2004, 143–44). The point is that an understanding of sex reflects a normative judgment that certain biological expressions and human actions are to be preferred over others.

Normative View of Disease

Paralleling this discussion, there is a prominent view in contemporary medicine regarding the *normative character of disease*. Contemporary physician-philosopher H. Tristram Engelhardt, Jr. (1981 [1975]) defends the view that disease is a normative concept that is to be understood in terms of harm or threat to well-being. It reflects a state of human dysfunction that is disvalued within a social context. "[E]valuation enters into the

enterprise of medical explanation because accounts of disease are imme-
diately focused on controlling and eliminating circumstances judged to be
of disvalue" (Engelhardt 1981 [1975], 137). The judgments are in no sense
pragmatically or performatively neutral. Choosing to call a set of phenomena "disease" involves a commitment to judging a clinical phenomenon to
be dysfunctional, enlisting the actions of health professionals, and intervening for purposes of achieving select goals.

Physician-philosopher Lawrie Reznek agrees with Engelhardt. Reznek
forwards the view that "[d]isease is to be understood in terms of the evaluative notion of being harmed." (1987, 170) For Reznek, "A has a disease P
if and only if P is an abnormal bodily/mental process that harms standard
members of A's species in standard circumstances" (1987, 162). Further,
"[s]omeone in state S has received harm if and only if he is worse off in state
S than he was before he was in state S" (1987, 136). Here, harm consists "in
the malfunction of systems worth having, or the frustration of worthwhile
pleasures, or the frustrations of worthwhile desires" (1987, 152). In the case
of having a disease, harm consists in the malfunction brought about by the
disease or the frustration brought about by the loss of worthwhile bodily
or mental desires. And these are not simply factual estimations about being
worse off; they are evaluative because they involve judgments concerning
what constitutes proper ends, form, and moral action.

The values that inform disease vary (Cutter 2003). Notions of good function surface in talk about effective organ, tissue, or cell action (Engelhardt
1996, 199–203). Because the measure of an organ (e.g., heart), tissue (e.g.,
cervical), or cell (e.g., pancreatic cell) is highly uninformative, a clinician has
no idea from just one single case what range of data can count as "normal"
and what can count as "abnormal." Group data is taken into account. What
is needed is a range of measurements for a range of populations that clinicians and researchers agree are diseased or healthy. Here "normal" can mean
that which is statistical, average or mean, typical or expectable, conducive to
the survival of a species, innocuous or harmless, commonly aspired to, and
excellent in its class (Murphy 1976, 117–33). In the case of gender-specific
disease, these measures quantify the processes through which gender-specific
factors contribute to the manifestation of disease. But these measures are not
value-neutral. The determination of what constitutes normal and pathological, and function and dysfunction, turns on a set of considerations regarding
what function is good and appropriate to the achievement of some ends,
goals, or purposes (also see Canguilhelm 1978 [1966]).

In addition, the medical goals of maximizing benefits (e.g., feeling good,
looking good, reducing pain) and minimizing harms (e.g., pain, inaccurate
diagnoses, high costs) involve instrumental values (Engelhardt 1996, 204).
In developing classifications for diseases, for instance, clinicians are concerned to minimize transaction and opportunity costs to the patient and
related parties (Cutter 1992). If one adopts standards for treatment that are
too lax, one may unduly increase the financial, social, and personal costs

for patients as well as society at large. However, if one sets the standards for treatment too strictly, one will pay the costs in the loss of lives. As a consequence, one must decide a prudent balancing of the transaction and opportunity costs related to over- and undertreatment. Such assessments turn on a set of considerations regarding what consequences or goals are worthy of achievement for the good or well-being of the patient.

Along with functional and instrumental values, aesthetic values operate in the framing of disease. Aesthetic judgments enter into how we understand disease in the sense that ideal states of physiological, anatomical, and psychological function presume a level of human ability, form, movement, and grace (Khushf 1999; Engelhardt 1981 [1975], 125). Judgments in medicine are aesthetic in that form and function are typically considered beautiful, and deformity and dysfunction ugly. Health typically correlates with form and function that is valued, and disease usually with form and function that is disvalued. Ideals of appearance and movement play an important role here. The kinds of form and function that are disvalued fail to meet ideals of symmetry, coherence, and visualization, as determined by patients as well as health care providers in particular communities and societies at large. Aesthetic judgments enter into how we frame gender-specific disease and emphasize properties that humans find aesthetically pleasing and displeasing.

Finally, disease involves choices (Engelhardt 1996, 226). One weighs the outcome of a process that has been brought to the attention of health care providers and the capacity to control the problem in a given situation involving particular patients against the harms that may be brought about by not acknowledging the process and not administering treatment. In other words, one must decide whether a clinical event is a gender-specific disease that is worth classifying, funding, diagnosing, and treating. In such cases, there are questions regarding who makes the choice and what choices ought to be made and why, who gets to assign and weigh the values at stake, and who is the ethical or moral authority in such situations. Typically in medicine, clinicians and researchers are granted the role and responsibility of classifying and describing gender-specific disease in part because of their familiarities with the methodologies employed and with what comes into the clinic. But patients have a role as well, as is evidenced by the role patient complaints play in framing disease diagnoses and treatments, despite medicine's move to replace the clinical encounter with technology and the laboratory. In this way, disease involves choices regarding what is good and proper function, what ends are to be sought, what is aesthetically pleasing, and what is the right thing to do.

Normative View of Disease Causation

The *causal relation between gender-specific factors and disease is normative* as well. In the previous section, a value-neutral account of causal relation understands the term "cause" to be used to identify conditions that are necessary to produce effects, sufficient to produce effects, or that contribute to the likelihood of an effect occurring. Whereas this approach in medicine involves great reliance on mathematical calculations, it does not follow that it is value-neutral. As Engelhardt argues, "[i]n the applied sciences, one is not interested simply in giving a coherent account [of the cause of disease], but in selecting among the possible coherent accounts those more useful in achieving one's goals and purposes. In most circumstances, it will not be worthwhile to attend to all the factors involved in giving a complete causal account. One directs one's attention and addresses instead those factors most easily manipulable" (1996, 223) (also see Agich 1997).

A manipulability account of causal relation holds that the way we pick out the most important cause is in terms of the manipulability of the various factors that lead to certain consequences (Collingwood 1940; von Wright 1971). In an early version of this account, philosopher G. von Wright (1971) describes the basic idea of the manipulability theory of causal relation as follows:

> [T]o think of a relation between events as causal is to think of it under the aspect of (possible) action. It is therefore true, but at the same time a little misleading to say that if p is a (sufficient) cause of q, then if I could produce p I could bring about q. For *that p* is the cause of q, I have endeavored to say here, *means* that I could bring about q, if I could do (so that) p (von Wright 1971, 74).

A cause, then, is that which one can manipulate in order to achieve a certain result. But what about those events which human beings cannot manipulate? Von Wright responds accordingly:

> The eruption of Vesuvius was the cause of the destruction of Pompeii. Man can through his action destroy cities, but he cannot, we think, make volcanos erupt. Does this not prove that the cause-factor is not distinguished from the effect-factor by being in a certain sense capable of manipulation? The answer is negative. The eruption of a volcano and the destruction of a city are two very complex events. Within each of them a number of events or phases and causal connections between them may be distinguished. For example, that when a stone from high above hits a man on his head, it kills him. Or that the roof of a house will collapse under a given load. Or that a man cannot stand heat above a certain temperature. All these are causal connections with which we are familiar from experience and which are such that the cause-factor typically satisfies the requirement of manipulability (von Wright 1971, 70).

Von Wright's view is that to understand a causal claim involving a cause that human beings cannot in fact manipulate (e.g., the eruption of a volcano), we must interpret it in terms of claims about causes that human beings *can* manipulate (e.g., impact of falling stones on human heads and so on).

Applied to our understanding the causal relation between gender-specific factors and disease, gender-specific factors represent those variables that can be manipulated in order to achieve the alleviation of suffering, pain, or dysfunction associated with disease. Of course, no one in gender-specific medicine is recommending a complete eradication or transformation of gender or sex in order to change disease conditions. No one is suggesting removing XX or XY chromosomes in an individual in order to change the course of a disease. This is practically and ethically not recommended. Rather, a focus in gender-specific medicine is to isolate which gender-specific factors that contribute to disease expression can be manipulated in order to change the condition of the disease. This is not simply a factual endeavor, it is an evaluative one. The determination of necessary, sufficient, and contributory causes of specific gender-specific diseases as well as what constitutes constantly conjoined events involves selecting out which variables can practically and ethically be manipulated for purposes of achieving selected goals. Choices are made about what options are practically possible and ethically permissible based on the taken-for-granted and expressed moral commitments.

VALUES, AND VALUES AND FACTS

One of the major sets of concerns lodged against a normative account of gender-specific disease draws our attention to the perils of relativism and the undermining of objectivity in medicine. More specifically, if values frame gender-specific disease, then the possibility of arriving at objective clinical descriptions and explanations of disease are severely threatened. We would not be able to maintain on medical grounds that X or Y gender-specific conditions were, or were not, diseases. We could only argue on social grounds that they *ought*, or ought not, to be *regarded* as diseases. As physician Robert Kendell puts the problem: "[W]e could not criticize Russian psychiatrists for incarcerating sane political dissidents in their beastly asylums [on medical grounds]: they would be perfectly entitled to regard political dissent as a mental illness if, as is probably the case, most of their fellow-citizens disapproved of political dissenters and it happened to be more convenient to deal with them as patients than as criminals" (Kendell 1971, 508). We could not criticize diagnosing slaves who run away from their masters with drapetomania (Cartwright 1981 [1851]), Wilson's account of menopause for its inaccurate overgeneralizations of menopausal women, and the early accounts of AIDS for their undergeneralizations of gender concerns as long as most people supported these views.

A charge of disease relativism often assumes that the values that frame disease are subjective. Here "subjective" means that which is based on someone's opinions or feelings rather than on facts or evidence. But what if the values that frame disease were objective? Philosopher Frederick Kaufman

(1997) argues that objective values secure the possibility of trans-cultural accounts of health and disease and prevent medical concepts from becoming relative (see also Pellegrino and Thomasma 1981). He elaborates on what he calls an objective account of disease normativism. For him, it is conceptually possible for normal function to count as disease, as in the case of cancer or heart disease among the elderly. Cancer and heart disease in the elderly can be considered normal biological events due to aging (see also Reznek 1987, 134–53; Goosens 1980, 106). Given this, malfunction or dysfunction cannot be a necessary condition for disease. Rather, harm, and not malfunction, is a necessary feature of disease (see also Reznek 1987; Engelhardt 1996, Ch. 5). It is the harm of a clinical condition that is the primary focus of medicine's efforts to understand and change a clinical condition. Such harm has to do with being "unable to exercise the capacities that constitute our good" (Kaufman 1997, 281). Through pharmaceutical, surgical, and palliative interventions, medicine offers the opportunity for patients to exercise such capacities, the normal range of which can be empirically established (Kaufman 1997, 281). Because harm is a necessary condition for disease, the objectivity of disease can be considered by way of the objectivity of harm. "If whether someone has been harmed is fixed by certain nonevaluative facts, such that one cannot accept those nonevaluative facts while denying harm, then harm can be an objective determination" (Kaufman 1997, 280). Because the concept of harm can be objectively defined, disease is not relative, as critics of disease normativism assume.

Kaufman's account of the objectivity of the values in disease saves a normativist account of disease from the problems of disease relativism. Gender-disease categories can be critiqued in light of how they satisfy clinico-scientific standards as well as how they benefit and/or harm patients. But one might ask about the defensibility of this objective account in light of the conclusions arrived at in the previous chapter, that an essentialist or traditionally speaking objective account of gender-specific disease is unavailable. If one understands Kaufman's sense of objectivity to refer to that which is universal, unchanging, and independent of the knower, then Kaufman's sense of objectivity is not defensible. As Chapter 2 has argued, humans do not have access to this kind of objective perspective and any suggestion that they do is misleading and can be harmful to patients.

If, however, one understands Kaufman's use of "objective" to refer to that which is shared, intersubjective, or able to be verified by means other than an omnipotent perspective (say, through an empirical or logical method and/or consensus), then Kaufman's sense of objectivity is compatible with a methodological naturalist view of gender-specific disease and the problem of gender-specific disease relativism is averted. But again, there is no suggestion that essentialist values will be able to be developed to guide and judge the development of gender-specific clinical classifications. We as humans simply do not have access to such knowledge.

Now that the role of values in gender-specific disease has been established, one might ask about the relation between facts and values in gender-specific disease. Are the facts and values operating in gender-specific disease separate and distinct? Here we return to the entailment gap and naturalistic fallacy mentioned earlier. Philosopher Philippa Foot (1958–59) helps us reflect on the question of their relation. Foot defends the view that facts are not as ontologically distinct from values as we have tended to assume in common discourse. She agrees that facts are not reducible to values (a form of strict prescriptivism [Hare 1952]), or values to facts (a form of strict naturalism [Perry 1954]). For Foot, if facts are reducible to values, then we are in the implausible position that anything at all can be counted as a "good reason" if we choose to make it a good reason. If values are reducible to facts, then we are in the implausible position that values such as choice and the good play no role in human life. For Foot, facts and values dually frame human life so that it makes no clear sense to distinguish them into two different types with different functions. Facts and values share action-guiding and factual features, such as found in the concept "dangerous." The word "dangerous" refers to threat that can be empirically confirmed as well as negatively judged. Threat can be empirically confirmed by observing it and gathering evidence to this effect. It can be negatively judged as evidenced by individual reports, means we take to prevent it, and reactions humans have to situations involving it. "Dangerous" is thus both factual and evaluative. Concepts like "dangerous" have so-called facts and values intertwined. The "factual" evidence that is given for threat involves negative judgments and reactions.

Foot's point is that facts are not so ontologically distinct from values. What one defines as a fact is a function of an empirical methodology. But the very selection of a fact can never be strictly empirical. What one singles out as worthy of pursuit and testing turns on judgments concerning what is of value, what has worth and should be pursued, and what lacks worth and should be avoided. What is selected as worthy of pursuit and attention is as much a function of evaluation as description. Thus, the line between facts and values, between description and prescription, is not so clear. A medical prescription that is offered by a clinician, for instance, is in part based on a judgment that a clinical condition is worthy of being treated, that there is something that a clinician can do about a clinical condition, and that a patient will be better off having been treated than not. But such a medical prescription is not recommended unless there is some evidence that it indeed has a chance of practically changing the clinical status of the patient and benefiting him or her. In other words, a medical prescription will not be said to be of value if it does not work.

It does not follow that there is no difference between facts and values. In the case of a prescription that is shown to work, lots of pharmaceutical agents affect the biological state of a patient, but the question is whether the pharmaceutical agent will benefit the patient. A cancer patient can experience change with chemotherapeutic drugs, antidepressants, or a massage, but what benefits the patient will turn on a host of considerations. If the patient has hopes for recovery, chemotherapeutic drugs may be advised. If the patient is terminal, pain medications, and not chemotherapeutic drugs, may be advised. What will benefit the patient turns on a host of judgments about clinical evidence made by an experienced clinician, the patient, and the patient's support group.

Applied to the concept of "gender-specific disease," gender-specific disease refers to facts about gender-specific disease as well as action-guiding judgments. More specifically, it refers to biological dysfunction explained via etiological laws, generalizations, or associations, and involves judgments that the biological dysfunction is disvalued and something should be done to change the condition. It involves a judgment to single out gender-specific conditions as opposed to non-gender-specific conditions for purposes of treating patients. In this way, gender-specific disease is both factual and evaluative.

SUMMARY

A *normative account of gender-specific disease* recognizes that gender, disease, and their relation are evaluative. It views gender-specific biological dysfunction explained via etiological laws, generalizations, or associations in terms of its role in providing treatment warrants. To select something as a gender-specific disease is to choose to single out certain evidence as worthy of attention, time, and funding. In this way, knowledge in gender-specific medicine is value-bound, centered as it is upon the phenomena of life, death, and human suffering. Cognitive claims in gender-specific medicine are judged in terms of their utility, their adaptive value, and their ability to satisfy human needs. Values and facts, evaluation and explanation, are twin endeavors in the process of describing and explaining gender-specific disease. Gender-specific disease is a "both/and" factual and evaluative concept in its meaning and use.

4 Gender-Specific Disease
Contextual Analysis

CONTEXTUALIZING CLINICAL PHENOMENA

Given that the concept of gender-specific disease describes and prescribes clinical reality within frameworks of understanding and evaluation, it follows that gender-specific disease is a contextual notion. The descriptive and prescriptive forces in gender-specific disease are backed by social sanctions, fashioned in light of what goals are seen to be worthy of achievement in our collective lives and located in nests of knowledge, actions, and settings. The question becomes, then, to what extent can gender-specific disease provide global accounts of clinical reality? Using the language found in the sociological literature, and adopting it to discussions of gender-specific disease, this chapter contrasts a *global* with a *local* account of gender-specific disease. The term "global" comes from the Latin term *globus*, which means "a ball or sphere," or pertaining to the earth. The term "local" comes from the Latin term *locus*, or "place." Whereas a global account of gender-specific disease spans beyond borders, a local account is constrained by borders. Because there are limits to both a global and a local account of gender-specific disease, the chapter argues in favor of a *trans-local account of gender-specific disease*. There is no timeless or essentialist account of gender-specific disease, or at least there is no such interpretation available to humans. Yet, given the methodological tools of medicine and our shared values, there are still ways in which we can classify and describe gender-specific disease.

THE FRAMES OF GENDER-SPECIFIC DISEASE

Roots of the appreciation of the historically and culturally conditioned character of knowledge are deep. Indeed, from the German philosophers G.W.F. Hegel (1777–1831) (1970 [1830]) and Ludwig Wittgenstein (1889–1951) (1963) to the present, there has been an increasing appreciation through the works of postmodernists, contextual epistemologists, and feminists of the extent to which our construals of reality exist within the embrace of cultural expectations. It was Hegel who recognized that the categories of knowledge as handed down by German philosopher

Immanuel Kant (1964 [1781/1787]) are historical. Kant held that we know reality through our concepts or categories of understanding. As he said, "what the things-in-themselves may be I do not know, nor do I need to know, since a thing can never come before me except in appearance" (Kant 1964 [1781/1787], 286). But Kant assumed that such categories of the understanding were ahistorical. Hegel's view was that the ways in which we see nature, and the concepts through which appearances are given to us, develop through time. As Hegel said: "By thinking things, we transform them [appearances] into something universal; things are singularities however, and the lion in general does not exist. We make them into something subjective, produced in us, belonging to us, and of course peculiar to us as men; for the things in nature do not think, and are neither representations nor thought" (Hegel 1970 [1830], 198, sec. 246, Zusatz). This view of understanding as a cultural endeavor is supplemented by Wittgenstein, whose claim about the relation between meaning and use and the multiplicity of "language games," each with its own set of norms, opened the way for a more thoroughgoing kind of semantic pluralism with regard to epistemic concepts and terms. As Wittgenstein said, "[e]ssence is expressed by grammar" (1963, sec 371); "[g]rammar tells us what kind of an object anything is" (1963, 373).

Contextual View of Gender and Sex

We'll begin our exploration of the contextual character of gender-specific disease with a consideration of the *contextual character of gender and sex*. Feminist philosopher Linda Alcoff (2006) argues that "gender is, among other things, a position one occupies and from which one can act politically" (Alcoff 2006, 148). She takes social position to foster the development of specifically gendered identities: "[T]he very subjectivity (or subjective experience of being a woman) and the very identity of women, are constituted by women's position" (Alcoff 2006, 148). She further holds that there is an objective basis for distinguishing individuals on the grounds of actual or expected reproductive roles: "*Women and men are differentiated by virtue of their different relationships of possibility to biological reproduction, with biological reproduction referring to conceiving, giving birth, and breast feeding, involving one's body*" (Alcoff 2006, 172, *italics in original*). Her view is that those standardly classified as biological female, even those who are unable to reproduce, will encounter "a different set of practices, expectations, and feelings in regard to reproduction than those standardly classified as male" (Alcoff 2006, 172). They experience a unique position with regard to reproduction that involves shared possibilities and reactions. This relation to reproduction is used as the basis for many cultural and social phenomena that position women as well as men. It often serves as "the basis of a variety of social segregations" (Alcoff 2006, 172) and fosters the construction and use of gendered social identities.

Because women are socially positioned in different cultural and experiential contexts, "there is no gender essence all women share" (Alcoff 2006, 147–48). Indian feminist philosopher Seemanthini Niranjana (2004) agrees: "Far from bearing a static meaning, the gender concept has aligned itself with a range of idea clusters from time to time, making it impossible to explain it by tracking its etymological roots alone" (Niranjana 2004, 137). Across the varied usages, and at the heart of the gender concept, has been attention to the manifestations and consequences of sexual differences in their cultural embeddedness. Whereas westerners often assume a notion of individuality as a basis of gender, non-westerners often assume a notion of social connectedness as the basis. Some see gender as primarily a scientific matter (Institute of Medicine 2001a), whereas others see it as a position of advocacy or political status (Cornell 2004). According to Niranjana, the gender debate concerns "how to understand differences—both between men and women, and among women themselves—suggesting that both biological and sociohistorical factors combine" (Niranjana 2004, 137; see entries in Tazi 2004).

Likewise, there is no sexual essence that all women share. Biologist Ruth Hubbard argues that "[w]omen's biology is a social construct and a political concept, not a scientific one" (2004, 65). She gives three reasons for holding this view. First, "female" and "male" are concepts that we grow up with, and the environment has significant influence on the ideas that we adopt. We are led to believe in a false dichotomy between gender and sex, and only with reflection can we begin to uncover the social forces that influence our supposedly scientific claims about femaleness and maleness. Second, female and male biologies are not simple facts out there to be discovered. They are the product of descriptions and explanations by others, and especially clinicians and scientists who adopt particular methods in order to generate knowledge claims. These methods are influenced by a host of forces, including social and political motives. One is reminded of claims made in the history of biology and medicine about the female body (see Tuana 1988, Ch. 1) that illustrate how agendas enter into how we know scientifically. Third, female and male biologies are "socially constructed and political because our society's interpretation of what is and is not normal and natural affects what we do" (Hubbard 2004, 66). Not only are our concepts and methods affected by outside forces, our very biologies are affected as well. One thinks here of how the foods we eat, the activities in which we engage, and the expectations of media and culture affect our biologies. Osteoporosis, for instance, is a consequence not simply of genetic endowment and calcium imbalance, but diets that limit calcium intake, a lifestyle that discourages weight-bearing exercises, and the social expectation to be thin. On this view, sex is not a pure scientific concept (see also Lorber and Moore 2002).

We are left with the recognition that gender and sex are contextual notions. As feminist sociologists Judith Lorber and Lisa Jean Moore say, "[n]either sex nor gender are pure categories. Combinations of genes, genitalia, and hormonal input are ignored in sexual categorization, just as combinations of incongruous physiology, identity, sexuality, appearance, and behaviors are ignored in the social construction of gender statuses" (Lorber and Moore 2002, 24). Menstruation, lactation, and gestation do not demarcate females from males, or women from men. Not all females/women have ovaries and uteruses. Only some females/women menstruate, only some lactate, only some become pregnant, and only some have ovaries and uteruses. Much depends on how the notions of gender and sex are framed, what constitutes the criteria, and for what purposes we use the categories.

Contextual View of Disease

In his book *Genesis and Development of a Scientific Fact*, physician-philosopher Ludwik Fleck (1979 [1935]) provides general guidance about how *disease is contextual*. Fleck argues that medical "facts" must be understood in terms of historical and psychosocial presuppositions. As the title of his book indicates, Fleck is concerned with the genesis and development of scientific facts, which are understood in terms of a particular *denkstil* or thought-style (Fleck 1979 [1935], 125–42), the carrier for the historical development of a given stock of knowledge and level of culture. They are understood as well in terms of a particular *denkkollectiv* or thought collective (Fleck 1979 [1935], 38–51), a community of persons mutually exchanging ideas or maintaining intellectual interaction. Fleck challenges the claim that "facts" are independent of the contexts in which they are fashioned. He embeds scientific thought and scientific facts in particular historical and societal contexts, thus continuing the Hegelian project of contextualizing knowledge, but in this case *medical* knowledge, and forecasting Thomas Kuhn's notable account of how paradigms operate in science (1996 [1962]).

Fleck elaborates his argument around a case study of syphilis. Syphilis, he argues, can be understood only if one assigns a temporal reference point indicating a particular thought-collective's or community's understanding of the disease. In the course of time, the character of syphilis changes from the mythical ("carnal scourge"), through the empirical and generally pathogenetical (with emphasis on clinical observation and experiment), to the mainly etiological (with the development of the Wasserman reaction). The transformation allows for "a rich resource of fresh details and a loss of seemingly irrelevant ones" (Fleck 1979 [1935], 19). It is brought about by more specific and reliable observations of the clinical condition as well as of the change in the clinical condition brought about by the use of therapeutic interventions, i.e., mercury followed by antibacteriological agents. Theoretical and practical elements, the *a priori* and *a posteriori* so to speak (Fleck 1979 [1935], 5), mingle with one another, thereby resulting in the clinical concept of "syphilis."

Psychiatrist George Engel also provides a contextual account of disease. Engel argues that the "biomedical" account of disease is mistaken. He contrasts a biomedical view of disease with what he calls a "biopsychosocial" view. A biopsychosocial view of disease contrasts with the biomedical model of disease presented in Chapter 2. A biopsychosocial view of disease holds that the presence of biochemical dysfunction is a necessary but not a sufficient condition for the occurrence of disease (Engel 1981 [1977], 595). It calls for further investigation of the role played by patient's symptomatic reports, the extent to which patient self-attribution of disease influences disease expression (597), how treatments work in light of a broader understanding of disease (597), and the influence of the care relation in the patient's healing process (597–98). It supports a scientific approach to behavioral and psychosocial phenomenon, including an assessment of the manifestation, onset, severity, and course of disease (597). But unlike a biomedical model, it portrays disease as biological dysfunction, loss of physical and mental integration, *and* loss of social networking. It resists reducing disease to the smallest discrete component having a causal biochemical variable outside the context of patient symptoms, the desires and goals of patients and health care providers, and social expectations and influences of a culture.

Physician-philosopher Lawrie Reznek (1987) offers a contemporary justification of a contextual account of disease. For him, contextualism characterizes "a domain of discourse where the truth of the sentences varies from one system to the next, because the sentences contain relational terms such that the truth conditions also vary from system to system" (Reznek 1987, 168). For example, anorexia nervosa is not a disease in a country in which food resources are seriously limited, but in a resource-rich environment. Sickle-cell trait is not pathological in malarial areas, but at high altitudes. Insensitivity to growth hormone is not a disease among pygmies, but one among the Masai. The point is that "[w]e cannot decide whether a judgment about disease-status is true without considering the relation of the condition to the organism, and the relation of the organism to the environment" (Reznek 1987, 169). One's disease may be another's adaptation to his or her environment.

A popular illustration of the contextual character of disease is found in examples of "culture-specific disease." "Culture-specific diseases" or "culture-bound syndromes" is a general term for certain psychiatric and psychological conditions and refer to recurrent, locality-specific patterns of aberrant behavior. Many of these patterns are indigenously considered to be "illnesses," or at least afflictions, and most have local names (Culture specific diseases 2007). An example of a culture-specific disease includes *amok* or *mata elap* from Malaysia, a dissociative episode characterized by a period of brooding followed by an outburst or violent, aggressive, or homicidal behavior. *Amok* is similar to *cafard* or *cathard* in Polynesia, *mal de pelea* from Puerto Rico, and perhaps "going postal" in American folk category. Other examples include *kuru*, a fatal disease of the brain and nervous system found among the South Foré people of the eastern New Guinea Highlands, and anorexia nervosa, an eating disorder that results in physical wasting seen in resource-rich western countries in which clean water and food are readily available. Culture-specific diseases appeal to non-allopathic criteria, such as myths drawn from folk psychology, in bringing the classification together. They are nevertheless considered very real to those in the particular culture in which it is expressed ("Culture specific diseases" 2007). They provide an example of diseases that are characterized by unique combinations of signs and symptoms, environmental circumstances, and cultural practices (Spector 1996).

Contextual View of Disease Causation

On a *contextual account*, how *gender-specific factors cause disease* depends on the factors that are deemed relevant in a system of thought. Revising a case from philosopher David Annis (1978, 215), suppose we are interested in whether Smith, a non-medical personnel, knows that HIV causes AIDS. If she responds that a pamphlet that she recently picked up at her local health fair says that it does, then we could claim that Smith knows that HIV causes AIDS. She has performed adequately given the context. But suppose the context is clinical experience. Suppose Dr. Wu in the early years of the AIDS epidemic reports a difference between the severity of HIV infection in a female and male at similar points in time of the progression of the disease. If infectious disease specialist Dr. Wu responds that her experience leads her to hold that HIV causes AIDS in a gender-specific way, we could say that she performed adequately given the context. Further suppose that the context is an examination for board certification in gender-specific medicine (something that is presently not available). Here we would expect much more. If the candidate, gender-specific specialist Dr. Moore, simply claims what Smith or Wu said, we might say that Dr. Moore does not know that HIV causes AIDS in a gender-specific way. Examiners would expect a detailed scientific elaboration of the differences between females and males, and how the manifestation, mechanism, and pharmaceutical treatment of AIDS vary as a function of HIV acting in different ways in females and males. Now, suppose an elected public health official, Mr. Calvin, claimed that "poverty, and not HIV, causes AIDS." Mr. Calvin is in some sense correct when it comes to the greater context of AIDS: that poverty leads to AIDS in females of resource-deprived regions in Africa in which females are sexually vulnerable. Yet, if this official were to answer on an examination for board certification in gender-specific medicine that poverty causes AIDS in females, the medical examiners would most likely claim that his answer was false based on the context in which the claim is made.

Put another way, a person S is justified in knowing P but not justified in knowing P relative to a system or context. The context determines the level of knowledge that S must exhibit. It determines what Annis (1978) calls the appropriate "objector-group" and the evaluation of the truth condition. It refers not to certain features of the object of knowledge but rather to features of the speaker's cognitive, psychological, and social situations. In the context of determining whether HIV causes AIDS, and in the context of expert knowledge, the appropriate objector-group is not the class of ordinary non-medical personnel or chair-side observers or elected officials, but rather qualified medical examiners in a particular field of study at a particular time and place. The appropriate objector-group is one who understands the intricacies of particular biological functioning and clinical practice. Other contextually relevant factors may enter in as well. These include the intentions, knowledge, beliefs, expectations, or interests of the speaker and audience; other speech acts that have been performed in the same context; time of utterance; effects of utterance; truth value of the proposition expressed; and semantic relations between the propositions expressed (Annis 1978). Although I will not review all of these here, the point is that situational, disciplinary, and other contextually relevant factors are an important part of the justification that a claim about disease causation is "true," for they in part determine what objections will be raised, how a knower will respond to them, and what responses the objectors will accept (also see Williams 1991; DeRose 1992; Cohen 1999).

LOCALIZING GENDER-SPECIFIC DISEASE

In order to understand gender-specific disease, then, one will have to learn the rules of evidence and inference accepted by those working in a particular community. One will have to understand how particular evaluative judgments regarding gender-specific disease frame the concept. One will, in addition, have to accept that our understanding of gender-specific disease evolves and changes with new knowledge and the recognition of previously unrecognized facts and values. Given the futility of discovering clinical reality fully, then, we begin to appreciate that *gender-specific disease is a local concept.*

Here "local" means particular or provisional as opposed to global or universal (Sassower and Cutter 2007, 62ff; Longino 1997). Gender-specific disease is local in terms of what and how it organizes knowledge claims. In a gender-specific medical context, AIDS, for instance, can be correlated with gender-specific genetic, immunological, and social variables, depending on whether one is a gender-specific molecular biologist, immunologist, or public health official. The construal will depend on the particular researcher's or clinician's appraisal of which gender-specific etiological variables operate in the framework the observer employs. For example, a gender-specific geneticist may attend to the role genetic factors that differ between members of particular sexes play in the transmission, reception, and processing of HIV. A gender-specific immunologist may decide that the major factor in AIDS is the lymphocyte count that differs between members of particular sexes. A gender-specific public health official may decide that the basic variables in AIDS are elements of a lifestyle that include unprotected sexual activities in a culture in which girls and women are most vulnerable. Gender-specific disease is "localized" or nested in particular systems of thought.

Further, our understanding of gender-specific disease influences and is influenced by how the condition is treated. Treatment will depend on the particular researcher's or clinician's appraisal of which gender-specific variables can best be manipulated. In the case of AIDS, a gender-specific geneticist may attend to how the genetic variables of the host and the virus can best be manipulated. A gender-specific immunologist may attend to how the lymphocyte count can be controlled and manipulated. A gender-specific public health official may seek to design political and economic initiatives that best target awareness of how HIV is transmitted in unprotected sexual encounters. There will be influences that affect the success of interventions that have more to do with the cultural acceptance of certain interventions. For instance, condoms will be accepted in cultures that accept medical advice on sexual matters, but not in ones in which medical advice is distrusted. Mandatory reporting of rape and incest in regions affected by AIDS will work in cultures that accept such reporting and not in one in which sexual matters are seen to be private or taboo. Treatment for gender-specific disease is "localized" insofar as it involves different accounts of what works depending on what can be manipulated and for what purposes.

Because all may not share the same view of a disease condition, one can expect disagreement about how to organize and employ gender-specific disease categories. One might recall the fervent debate in the early 1990s regarding how AIDS might be gender-specific. The first natural history study of HIV disease in women began in 1992 (Landesman and Holman 1995), and it was in 1993, ten years after AIDS was first reported in women, that the CDC first publicly recognized that HIV-related symptoms specific to women existed (Corea 1992, 346). In 1992, the agency modified its surveillance definition of AIDS by adding invasive cervical cancer to the list of AIDS-defining conditions, along with pulmonary tuberculosis and recurrent pneumonia (Centers for Disease Control 1992). Conditions that were manifested most frequently in HIV-infected women (such as recurrent vulvovaginal candidiasis, pelvic inflammatory disease, and cervical dysplasia) became part of the list of "symptomatic conditions in an HIV-infected adolescent or adult" (although one might note that they were not included among conditions listed as "AIDS-defining") (Centers for Disease Control 1992). In 1996, still only an estimated 1% of the AIDS literature focused on women-specific manifestations of the disease (Faden et al. 1996). By 2006, the number of people living with HIV/AIDS climbed to 33.2 million worldwide, 15.4 million of whom were women and 2.5 million of whom were children. By 2006, more than twenty-five million people worldwide had died of AIDS since 1981 and Africa reported twelve million AIDS orphans. At the end of 2006, females accounted for 50% of all adults living with HIV worldwide and for 61% in sub-Saharan Africa (Worldwide HIV and AIDS 2007). And yet, the diagnosis and treatment of AIDS worldwide continues to be rather gender-neutral. Differences in how gender-specific disease is understood lead to differences in gender-specific disease taxonomies.

GLOBALIZING LOCAL ACCOUNTS

In light of the recognition that gender-specific disease is a local concept, we are left with questions about the possibility of developing stable, enduring nosologies and nosographies for gender-specific disease. Although philosophical reasons for rejecting a universal account of gender-specific disease have been given, what about the more practical issues concerning our capacity to talk about gender-specific disease on a scale that goes beyond local borders? Are we left with an inability to speak beyond boundaries and borders? How might we respond to the efforts of the World Health Organization (WHO) and the United Nations (UN), both of which appear to forward *a global account of gender-specific disease*?

By way of background, the World Health Organization (WHO) has developed a Department of Gender, Women, and Health (GWH) to bring "attention to the ways in which biological and social differences between women and men affect health and the steps needed to achieve health equity" (Department of Gender, Women, and Health 2007, 1). Though gender affects the health of both women and men, the GWH places emphasis on the health consequences of discrimination against women that exist in nearly every culture. Influential barriers, including poverty, unequal power relationships between women and men, and lack of education, prevent millions of women worldwide from having access to health care and from attaining and maintaining the best possible health. The GWH's main areas of work in the new millennium include violence against women and its effect on women's health, HIV/AIDS (e.g., the development of guidelines for gender-sensitive HIV/AIDS programs), and the integration of gender into health policies and programs (e.g., the assessment of gender differences and inequalities in the planning, implementation, monitoring, and evaluation of WHO's work).

A major goal of such programming is gender-mainstreaming, which the UN defines as "a globally accepted strategy for promoting gender equity" (United Nations 2008b, 1). Here, gender refers to "the social attitudes and opportunities associated with being male and female and the relationships between women and men and girls and boys, as well as the relations between women and those between men" (United Nations 2008a, 1). Gender equality "refers to equal rights, responsibilities, and opportunities of women and men and boys and girls. Equality does not mean that women and men will become the same but that womens [sic] and mens [sic] rights, responsibilities, and opportunities will not depend on being born male and female" (United Nations 2008a, 1). Mainstreaming involves ensuring that "gender perspectives and attention to the goal of gender equality are central to all activities—policy development, research, advocacy/dialogues, legislation, resource allocation, and planning, implementation, and monitoring of programmes and projects" (United Nations 2008b, 1). Gender-mainstreaming involves, then, the means of integrating gender concerns into the analysis, formulation, and monitoring of health programs and projects with the objective of ensuring that inequalities between women and men are reduced, if not eradicated.

Few would argue that the goal of developing ways to understand biological and social differences between women and men that affect health is not worthwhile. To begin with, we already communicate across borders and locales about gender-specific disease conditions and health challenges faced by women. Shared here in our communication will be clinical evidence of disease conditions and their challenges. Shared here will also be claims and values concerning what clinical "circumstances are likely to be impediments to the realization of goals (1) in nearly every foreseeable environment and (2) in terms of any likely cluster of human purposes" (Engelhardt 1996, 204). These likely will include ones related to living a secure life and having access to food, shelter, income, medical care, and transportation.

In light of the conclusions arrived at in our investigation so far, how can we recognize the limits of a local account of gender-specific disease while at the same time secure the possibility of talking about gender-specific clinical issues that need attention worldwide? If the WHO and UN use "global" to mean universal or essential, or that there is *a* way of understanding and treating gender-specific disease, then the argument has already been given for why a global account of gender-specific disease is unavailable. To conclude otherwise would be to disregard the conclusions of earlier discussions regarding the contextuality of describing and prescribing gender-specific disease. A global account is unavailable because gender-specific descriptions and prescriptions depend on the rules of evidence and inference accepted by those working in a particular community, which evolve and change with new knowledge and the recognition of previously unrecognized facts and values.

If, however, the WHO and UN understand "global" in a non-universalist or non-essentialist way, in a way that conveys the idea of a generalized view of human experience and one that indicates shared knowledge and value claims within specified contexts, then a global account of gender-specific disease will be available. The challenge in medicine will be to remain vigilant in appreciating the nuances in our languages and perspectives, differences in our bodies that are a function of environmental forces, and variations in our collective medical practices. As Margaret Urban Walker put the problem of our developing "imagined" (or in our case imagined "global") communities, "[i]magined communities are seductive because they yield real psychic comforts, powerful feelings of belonging and mattering; imagined communities are irrelevant or dangerous because they distract our attention from actual communities" (Walker 1994, 54). In the case of gender-specific disease, we can find shared knowledge about how women can be harmed. We can also find shared concerns about what goals are worthy to be pursued and which ones hinder the pursuit of the good. Attending to the nuances in language and perspective, bodily and psychic differences, and differences in accepted medical practices will be critical to the success of any global perspective on gender-specific disease. Otherwise, the global perspective will fail to meet the needs of actual patients and it may, in fact, harm patients if ideology, as opposed to critical deliberation, takes over.

A *trans-local account of gender-specific disease* provides ways to bridge shared notions about sexual and gender status, disease predicament, and their relation. We can talk locally at global levels about gender-specific disease that in our clinical experience create fruitful discussions and interventions that help individuals, tribes, communities, and societies achieve their goals. There will be small-scale agreement, as may be found in cases of gender-specific culture-bound diseases and their recommended treatments, as well as wide-spread agreement, as might be found in the case of diagnosing gender-specific heart disease. There will be volatile debate, as may be found in discussions concerning proper nomenclature for disorders of sex development, and milder debates, as may be found in discussions concerning the need for better diagnostics for gender-specific heart disease. The concept of gender-specific disease can be attentive to shared notions of gender, disease, and their relation, and yet accommodate differences across local communities and cultures. The shared notions will depend on agreement about the method used to determine clinical evidence, the desired goals, and ways to interpret them. Differences will emerge, as methods, goals, and interpretations vary.

SUMMARY

A *trans-local account of gender-specific disease* recognizes that gender, disease, and their relations are nested within frames of reference. Gender-specific disease contextualizes how we understand gender-specific biological dysfunction explained via etiological laws, generalizations, or associations for purposes of providing treatment warrants. Whereas gender-specific disease is "local" in the sense in which it has particular expressions depending on the context, it is "global" in the sense that there are shared views of gender, disease, and their relation made possible by the tools of medicine, the ways humans interpret, and the goals humans seek to achieve. Gender-specific disease is "both/and" global and local in its meaning and use.

5 An Integrative Approach to Gender-Specific Disease

DESCRIBING AND PRESCRIBING IN SOCIAL CONTEXTS

This chapter bridges what in the last three chapters has been separated. It brings the discussions of Chapters 2 through 4 together and calls for *an integrative approach to understanding gender-specific disease.* Here the term "integrative" comes from the Latin *integratus*, which means "to make whole." Using the language of integrative clinicians, and adopting it to discussions of gender-specific disease, it draws from the works of integrative physicians Andrew Weil (1995, 2004) and Christiane Northrup (2002) and develops their thinking with the philosophical and sociological contributions of intersectional health sociologists Amy L. Schulz and Leith Mullings (2006) and Chloe Bird and Patricia Rieker (2008). An integrative approach sees gender-specific disease as biological dysfunction brought about by gender-specific factors explained via etiological laws, generalizations, or associations within particular historical and cultural frameworks for purposes of developing treatment warrants. Approaching gender-specific disease integratively assists in highlighting the mutually constitutive roles that description and prescription play in situating gender-specific disease.

CONNECTING THE FOREGOING

Consider the interconnectedness among the multiple dimensions of gender-specific disease presented in Chapters 2 through 4. In terms of description, and as Chapter 2 illustrates, gender-specific disease is in part discovered and in part created. It is discovered in the sense that gender-specific disease is a product of nature, where nature is understood not simply as a thing out there to be discovered, separate and distinct from human knowers, but rather as the source, substance, and process of all living beings (Bender 2003, 20). Gender-specific disease is created in the sense that sex and gender are more complex than a discoverable, binominal, fixed, and discrete category of nature, and disease is more than discoverable biological dysfunction. Further, the relation between sex/gender and disease defies being reduced to a single causal relation. Gender-specific disease is multi-factorial and involves a host of biological and environmental factors understood within the context of certain settings. Gender-specific disease is an expression of the limits of nature and the lenses we bring to such expressions. In this way, gender-specific disease is a methodological naturalist concept.

In this process of description and explanation, and as Chapter 3 argues, gender-specific nosologies and nosographies give rise to the development of norms. Such norms function prescriptively; they serve as the basis for judgments about how individuals of a certain sex with certain conditions ought to be and to act, including being pain-free and able to pursue life's goals. Ideals of activity and those of form and grace that are proper to an organism are brought to bear on such judgments. Further, we decide how to act, what to strive for, and what to resist in light of such norms. If one conforms to gender-specific disease norms, one increases the probability of being a recipient of clinical intervention and social support. If one diverges from such norms, one lessens the chance of being recognized as a recipient of clinical intervention and social support. Gender-specific disease is a cluster of characteristics and abilities that function as standards by which individuals of a certain sex/gender and their conditions are judged to be "good" or "bad" instances of particular ideals of human function or ability. In this way, gender-specific disease is a normative concept.

Alternatively, norms give rise to clinical descriptions and explanations. What and how humans value and disvalue influence what presents in the clinical curricula and textbooks, what is funded in clinical research, and what becomes foci of attention in local and national health policies. Individuals, communities, and institutions rally around what is seen to be worthwhile targets of attention in health care, thereby encouraging the allocation of time, talent, and funds toward particular clinical endeavors which can result in new knowledge in clinical medicine. At the same time, individuals, communities, and institutions resist pursuing what may be seen to be less-than-worthwhile avenues of pursuit, thereby discouraging time, talent, and funding toward other knowledge endeavors in clinical medicine. Either way, evaluations in part guide what descriptions and explanations gender-specific medicine adopts because they determine what will and what will not be worthy of attention.

As framed here, the descriptive level of analysis of gender-specific disease intersects with the prescriptive. Facts and values, and theory and practice, interplay in complex ways. Observations in gender-specific medicine are always ordered around theoretical commitments, including judgments concerning how to select and organize evidence into descriptions and explanations. Further, observations are always ordered around evaluative commitments, including those concerning what phenomena are assigned significance in terms of what actions are appropriate in order to achieve select goals. Use of the term "gender-specific disease" reflects a choice to emphasize the gender-specific components of disease and to de-emphasize non-gender-specific ones which operate as well. It involves a practical commitment to pursue a certain line of study over another. It requires the allocation of resources and entails the motive to help patients find relief from the pain and suffering associated with gender-specific dysfunction. Observations in gender-specific medicine are themselves instruments of human adaptation and the value of cognitive claims are judged in terms of their utility, their adaptive value, and their ability to satisfy human needs. In this way, knowing clinical reality is never a purely theoretical endeavor but a form of practice or, as philosopher Marx Wartofsky (1975, 188) calls it, *praxis*, an endeavor of doing and making. It involves "rich, historical contexts of fundamental and even revolutionary modes of cognitive praxis" (Wartofsky 1976, 188).

The descriptive and prescriptive forces in gender-specific medicine are nested in particular contexts and framed in terms of individual, communal, and societal goals. These goals turn on the rules of evidence and inference accepted by those working in particular communities. In gender-specific medicine, the rules often relate to how one weighs the outcomes of a process that have been brought to the attention of health care professionals and the capacity to control the problematic process experienced by a patient or group of patients against the harms that may be brought about by not acknowledging the process and not administering treatment. Such rules of evidence and inference evolve and change with new knowledge and technology and the recognition of previously unrecognized valued and disvalued states of affairs. The rules of evidence and inference depend not only on the methodological assumptions of the clinical method but on socio-economic factors. In this way, gender-specific disease is a trans-global concept.

In short, the multiple dimensions of gender-specific disease do not operate alone but rather interplay in various and complex ways. Description and prescription, facts and values, and theory and practice mutually define and situate each other within particular contexts.

TOWARD AN INTEGRATIVE APPROACH TO GENDER-SPECIFIC DISEASE

The analysis put forth in this project leads us to embrace what I call an *integrative approach* to gender-specific disease. The initial inspiration for this approach is taken from integrative medicine and the works of physicians Andrew Weil (1995) and Christiane Northrup (2002). "Integrative" or "holistic" medicine entails a balanced, whole-person-centered approach to health care and involves a synthesis of conventional or allopathic medicine, complementary and alternative modalities, and/or traditional medical systems, with the aim of prevention and health as a basic foundation. It is to be distinguished from non-synthetic approaches such as "unorthodox" medicine, "alternative" medicine, and "complementary" medicine that may seek to operate alone separate from conventional or allopathic medicine (Lee et al. 2004, 10; Weil 1995; Kligler and Lee 2004). Although integrative medicine may at this point in time be more of an ideal than a practical reality, it is worth considering for how it supports the conclusions thus far in this analysis and provides guidance for the practice of gender-specific medicine.

Integrative medicine gained momentum in the U.S. toward the end of the twentieth century. Socio-political movements such as the civil rights, women's rights, consumer rights, and wellness movements supported changes in medicine that empowered patients as decision-makers and active participants and encouraged a move away from seeing the patient as an object. In 1993, the National Institutes of Health opened the Office of Alternative Medicine, which was later renamed in 1998 as the National Center for Complementary and Alternative Medicine (NCCAM) (2009). The NCCAM is the Federal Government's lead agency for scientific research on the diverse medical and health care systems, practices, and products that are not generally considered part of conventional or allopathic medicine. It received $121,577,000 in public funding for fiscal year 2008. In 2007, consumers spent $33.9 billion in out-of-pocket expenses on complementary and alternative medicine, a figure that reflects 1.5% of total health care expenditure in the U.S. and 11.2% of the total of out-of pocket health care expenses (National Center for Complementary 2009).

In 1997, physician Andrew Weil started the first fellowship program in integrative medicine at the University of Arizona Medical School. Today, there are a number of integrative programs in medical schools and centers around the country. Data from 2004 show that 36% of adults used some form of complementary and alternative treatment to manage their health (Rakel and Weil 2007). A landmark publication by health economist David Eisenberg and colleagues in 1993 revealed that the public was spending $13 billion dollars out of pocket for CAM. A subsequent study, published five years later, showed a similar trend with an even higher percentage (42%) of Americans using CAM in 1997 and out-of-pocket expenditures for CAM increasing by 27% over the earlier study (Eisenberg et al. 1998). The use of complementary and alternative treatment in medicine continues to increase today.

Generally put, integrative medicine rejects defining human disease and patients along the lines found in a biomedical account, namely in an objective, reductionistic, positivist, and determinist manner (Koopsen and Young 2009, xvii). Here, for the integrative practitioner, "objectivity" entails that the observer is separate from the observed and the observer can fully know the observed, as in the case of seeing a patient's disease as distinct from the patient, the disease and the patient as "objects," and the health care provider as an objective observer of the patient. "Reductionism" occurs when complex phenomena are simply explained by component phenomena, as seen in the case of understanding AIDS simply as HIV. "Positivism" means that information is derived strictly from physically measurable data, as is the trend in contemporary medicine with its

reliance on laboratory data, as opposed to patient complaints, to understand a disease finding. "Determinism" occurs when phenomena are pre-
dicted from knowledge of scientific law and initial conditions and given
more predictive power that is warranted, as suggested in the statements
"It's in the gene" or "The gene for . . .".

In contrast, integrative medicine seeks to include a partnership between
patient and practitioner in the healing process and to use conventional
and alternative methods to facilitate the body's natural healing process.
It involves a consideration of the many factors that influence health and
disease, including mind, body, and spirit, and thereby rejects a reductionist
view of human disease. It supports a philosophy that neither rejects conventional medicine nor accepts alternative therapies uncritically. It recognizes
that good medicine needs to be based in good science, be inquiry-driven,
and be open to new paradigms, but not without acknowledging the role
patient reporting plays in determining diagnosis and treatment. In this way,
integrative medicine rejects a simple positivist and determinist approach to
disease. It encourages patients to talk with their clinicians and clinicians
to spend time interviewing their patients. It uses natural, effective, multi-
factorial interventions whenever possible, and involves broader concepts of
the promotion of health and the prevention of illness as well as the treatment of disease (Arizona Center 2009).

Integrative researchers John Astin and Kelly Forys (2004, 34) call for an
integrative approach to understanding and treating disease. This includes
using the thinking and treatments from traditional medical systems such
as biomedical or allopathic medicine as well as Ayurveda, Chinese, East
Asian, and Native American medicines. It also includes manual medicines such as osteopathy and chiropracty; lifestyle interventions such as
diet and exercise; mind-body interventions such as hypnosis, biofeedback,
and spiritual interventions; botanical medicines such as herbs; and energy
medicine such as homeopathy and reiki. A goal here is to understand disease not as a thing out there to be discovered, but rather as a process of
the body, mind, and spirit that signals a need for change and rebalance.
A goal as well is to find treatments that are safe and effective for patients
based on both allopathic and non-allopathic principles, keeping in mind
that the patient's body, mind, and spirit hold the recipes for treatment and
guidelines to healing.

As an illustration, compare an allopathic with an integrative approach
to premenstrual syndrome (PMS). For the allopathic clinician, PMS is a
condition of recurrent physical and psychological symptoms, occurring in
a cyclic fashion during the one- to two-week period preceding a woman's
menstrual period, significant enough to cause disruption in either family,
personal, or occupational function (Girman et al. 2004, 763). Premenstrual syndrome (PMS) appears to be caused by multiple endocrine factors
(e.g., hypoglycemia, other changes in carbohydrate metabolism, hyperpro-
lactinemia, fluctuations in levels of circulating estrogen and progesterone,

abnormal responses to estrogen and progesterone, and excessive aldosterone [ADH]). Estrogen and progesterone can cause transitory fluid retention, as can excess ADH. "In its most severe form, it [PMS] affects roughly 2.5% of women of reproductive age; in a more mild form, it is estimated to affect approximately 40% of women in this age group" (Girman et al. 2004, 763). In allopathic medicine, a wide range of pharmaceutical approaches are used to treat the symptoms of PMS, including oral contraceptives and other hormonal supplements, non-steroidal antiinflammatories, bromocriptine, and diuretic agents. Most recently, antidepressants, particularly the selective serotonin reuptake inhibitors, have become popular for women who struggle with depression or mood instability.

Integrative approaches to PMS understand PMS in a broader sense. PMS is not simply a biochemical imbalance within the patient but an indication of lifestyle imbalance. Integrative diagnostics focus on the broad array of factors that contribute to hormonal imbalance and subsequent PMS symptoms. Integrative treatments involve a variety of approaches and include nutritional approaches, botanical medicine, and exercise (e.g., yoga, aerobic exercise), manipulative therapy (e.g., massage), and homeopathy. Nutritional approaches include dietary manipulation such as the removal of dairy products, refined sugars, and high-sodium foods and caffeine intake in the diet (Girman et al. 2004, 764). Magnesium, vitamin B6, calcium supplements, and botanical medicines, such as chastetree (vitex), black cohosh, St. John's wort, kava, and ginko (Girman et al. 2004, 764–68), may be recommended. Yoga and aerobic exercise contribute to the reduction of stress in a patient's life (Girman et al. 2004, 766). The integrative practitioner's job is to help orchestrate the care of patients in light of the biopsychosocial factors contributing to the patient's disease or illness in order to maximize the benefits of treating patients.

Further, and relevant to our investigation of gender-specific disease, integrative physician Christiane Northrup (2002) helps us think through how medicine genders disease through her work with women. In addressing the character of disease, Northrup notes that contemporary western medicine describes bodies "not as natural systems homeostatically designed to tend toward health but rather as war zones" (Northrup 2002, 8). Contemporary medical preferences for drugs and surgery as treatments are part of what she calls an "aggressive patriarchical" (Northrup 2002, 8) approach to disease. In our aggressive hierarchy, "our society demands that women, its second-class citizens, ignore or turn away from their hopes and dreams in deference to men and the demands of their families" (Northrup 2002, 6). It assumes that disease is the enemy (Northrup 2002, 7) and medical science is omnipotent (Northrup 2002, 9). It assumes that patients cannot possibly know more about their clinical conditions, and women's normal life experiences, such as PMS, menstruation, pregnancy, and menopause, require medical attention, and specifically pharmaceuticals. Although Northrup recognizes that short-term remedies such as drugs may be beneficial, she

calls for recasting disease in terms of a "messenger trying to get our attention" (Northrup 2002, 8) and of the body as the best guide to healing. She
demonstrates through her work with women that when women change the
basic conditions of their lives that lead to health problems, they heal faster,
more completely, and with far fewer medical interventions (Northrup 2002,
Chs. 2 and 3, 25ff).

Consider Northrup's discussion of PMS (2002, 129–40) and how this
extends the earlier integrative approach to PMS by addressing more specifically how medicine genders disease. Northrup begins by saying that
"[n]o modern disorder points to the need to rethink our ideas about
menstruation and reclaim the wisdom of our cycles more directly than
the common malady known as premenstrual syndrome, or PMS. Having
treated hundreds of women with PMS, I know that such a rethinking is
needed to get to the root causes of PMS" (Northrup 2002, 129). Although
Northrup recommends dietary changes, exercise, vitamins, and progesterone therapy in treating PMS, she calls for a look at the imbalances that
exist that biochemical changes alone cannot help. "As studies have confirmed, unresolved emotional problems may disrupt the menstrual rhythm
and the normal hormonal milieu" (Northrup 2002, 129). She states that
the many symptoms associated with PMS are related to eicosanoid imbalances that result from a complex interaction of emotional and social factors (Northrup 2002, 130). Though some doctors are still looking for a
"biochemical lesion" that "causes" PMS, no one has been able to find a
lesion or a magic bullet to cure it (Northrup 2002, 131–32). "A reductionistic approach—looking for the chemical 'cause' and 'cure'—simply
doesn't work because the causes of PMS are multifactorial and must be
approached holistically. The effects of the mind, emotions, diet, light,
exercise, relationships, heredity, and childhood traumas must all be taken
into account when treating PMS" (Northrup 2002, 132). Many women
are given symptomatic treatments for PMS that over the long run do not
work. Treating a woman's bloating with diruretics, her headaches with
painkillers, her cramps with oral contraceptives, and her anxiety with
the antidepressant Valium often serve to create new side effects from the
drugs themselves and ignore the underlying imbalances that led to PMS
in the first place (Northrup 2002, 135).

Taken together, Weil and Northrup give us insight into how to approach
gender-specific disease integratively. Some of the current research on gender-specific disease currently assumes that gender variations in disease are
due strictly to underlying biological difference, that they convey clear lines
of difference between members of different genders, and that medicine will
be able to provide accounts of how gender-specific factors directly cause
disease (see Chapter 1). An integrative approach challenges these taken-for-
granted notions in medicine and provides practical guidance in navigating
the interrelations among the descriptive, prescriptive, and contextual roles
of gender-specific disease.

INTERSECTIONS BEYOND GENDER AND DISEASE

Heeding the lessons of an integrative approach to gender-specific disease, we are reminded that gender-specific factors are not the only causal variables in gender-specific disease. Gender does not operate alone, but rather intersects with other categories of analysis that contribute to disease. These include, among others, race, ethnicity, class, socio-economic status, age, and other dimensions of influence and difference. This type of "intersectional" thinking arises out of the work of feminists over the last few decades (Crenshaw 1991; Collins 2000) and focuses on the relations among gender, sexuality, race/ethnicity, class, and other dimensions of influence and difference. Kimberlé Williams Crenshaw (1991) introduced the idea of "intersectionality" to demonstrate how race, class, and gender are all part of how black women live their blackness and their womanhood and how they are discriminated against in society through the interaction of these three forms of oppression (Cornell 2004, 38). Intersectionality demands that those working with the concept of gender expand the analysis of gender. The category of "gender" no longer singly names a social identity; it intersects with other categories of analysis and dimensions of influence and difference. Gender becomes a process of social relations and not simply a biological "fact" of an individual, patient, or subject.

Applied to our understanding of gender-specific disease, one will not be fully able to understand the role of gender in disease if one does not also investigate how gender is classed, raced, ethnicized, aged, and so on. An intersectional approach to disease views disease as embedded within "processes through which multiple social inequalities of gender, race, ethnicity, social class, and other dimensions of difference are simultaneously generated, maintained, and challenged at institutional and individual levels, shaping the health of societies, communities, and individuals" (Weber 2006, 25). Although this is a demanding request, it philosophically makes great sense in light of the findings in the previous chapters. It also makes practical sense in terms of the research offered by intersectional health researchers.

Health sociologists Leith Mullings and Amy Schulz (2006, 5–6) encourage medicine to examine the ways in which gender, race, and class are mutually defining so that we can further break down problematic conceptions of the category of "gender" and offer ways to approach disease found in medicine. Current medical research attends mostly to variations in disease by single causal categories (e.g., gender, race/ethnicity, or class) as opposed to their intersections. For sure, traditional methods of investigation typically found in biomedical research have been useful in forming and testing predictive models in which the emphasis is on independent, discrete variables within epidemiological models. But, according to intersectional researchers Pamela Braby Jackson and David R. Williams (2006), health researchers seldom consider how disease is distributed when three or more social status categories are considered simultaneously. In light of this sort of problem, Jackson and Williams (2006) uncover what they call the *intersectionality paradox*. This paradox "captures the recurring dilemma of certain health problems faced at the intersection of race, SES [socio-economic status], and gender by members of the black middle class" (Jackson and Williams 2006, 138).

Jackson and Williams (2006) show how, at the intersection of race, class, and gender, new experiences emerge that undermine the benefits of being a member of the black middle class. African American middle-class women, for instance, are disadvantaged on a variety of health outcomes. "In national data, the highest SES group of African American women has equivalent or higher rates of infant mortality, low birth weight, hypertension, and excess weight than the lower SES group of white women" (Jackson and Williams 2006, 139). Citing Elsie Pamuk et al. (1988), they show that African American women are more than twice as likely to suffer the loss of an infant than their non-Hispanic white counterparts. Further, the black-white differential in infant mortality becomes larger as maternal education increases (Jackson and Williams 2006, 142). Among whites, women who did not complete high school have an infant mortality rate that is 2.4 times the rate of women who graduated from college. Similarly, among African Americans, women with less than twelve years of education have an infant mortality rate that is 1.5 times as high as that of college graduates (Jackson and Williams 2006, 142).

Consider what an intersectional approach to smoking-related lung cancer adds to our understanding and treatment of a gender-specific problem. A traditional method of investigation might involve determining what about the biology of a woman leads her to develop smoking-related lung cancer at a faster rate than a man. It is becoming well established that women are more vulnerable to tobacco toxins than men and that women are 1.3 to 2.9 times more likely to develop lung cancer than men (Haugen 2002, 227). Although this evidence is critically important in understanding gender-specific lung cancer, it is insufficient for developing treatment recommendations for gender-specific lung cancer. Intersectional theorist Lynn Weber (2006, 37–39) explores the power relationships that shape those who smoke, why they smoke, and how their smoking is interpreted by others. She draws from Oaks (2001), who documents that poor and working-class women are more likely to smoke during pregnancy and to be labeled unfit and irresponsible mothers when they do because this image reinforces dominant-cultural conceptions of their communities. Critical institutional and interpersonal power relationships shape the contexts of the lives of women, producing stresses and constraints for which smoking provides relief.

Further, with regard to treatment, it is typical to see the claim that those who smoke are weak in some sense and require individual intervention to assist in "kicking the habit" through individual smoking cessation programs (Lancaster et al. 2002). Indeed, smoking prevention and cessation programs have been extensively tested in experimental studies in industrialized countries (Lancaster et al. 2002). But there is little data that shows that this approach works in other settings, much less data showing differences in how women and men respond to particular styles of intervention. Bhutta et al. (2003, in Mullings and Schulz 2006) reported that less than 5% of all randomized trials and systematic reviews of interventions were based on investigations in representative community settings. Given that an average of 22% of individuals worldwide smoke, that many more experience second-hand smoking, and that smoking correlates with lung and respiratory problems, one can conclude that there is a large body of knowledge regarding patient health that is missing in public health initiatives in global medicine. Treatments for lung problems, such as ensuring access to a living wage, health care insurance and delivery, preventive health care, quality education, and safe and affordable housing, are often not considered options in smoking-prevention initiatives. Given women and men have a disproportionate level of access to such opportunities in certain settings, questions remain as to the effectiveness of treatment programs.

An intersectional approach to gender-specific disease gives insight into the interaction between gender and other dimensions of analysis in disease expression and treatment. In particular, it examines the ways in which gender, race/ethnicity, class, age, and other dimensions of difference are mutually constitutive and interconnected and, ultimately, how those interconnections work to produce gender-specific clinical conditions and to guide treatment recommendations.

A FURTHER WORD ON RACE AND CLASS

I would be remiss if I did not address some of the concerns that have been raised about the use of the concepts of race and class in medicine. I will share a few thoughts concerning the special challenges of investigating race and class as contributing factors of disease and show the relevancy of these concerns to challenges in framing gender-specific disease. By singling out race and class, I do not mean to undermine the previous conclusion that it is important to consider the mutually constitutive and interconnected factors that contribute to disease. In addition, I do not mean to underemphasize the role of age and other dimensions of influence and difference in the analysis of gender-specific disease. My point is to show that, as is the case in its use of gender, medicine will need to be careful in its use of other factors of influence and difference in disease expression.

A first concern has to do with the problem of ambiguity of the concepts of race and class in medicine. The historically contingent character of racial categories highlights their changing socially and politically constructed nature. Consider a brief recounting from history. In 1790, the U.S. Census Bureau adopted three categories: Free Persons (white, and all other free persons except Indians not taxed), slaves (counted as three-fifths of a person), and Indians living on reservations (not taxed). By 1850, categories shifted to more explicit racial language denoting simply white and free persons of color. By 1890, an expanded range of racial categories included white, black (persons with three-quarters or more "black blood"), mulatto (one-half black ancestry), quadroon (one-fourth black ancestry), and octoroon (one-eighth black ancestry). By 1910, these categories aggregated the previous distinctions in percentage ancestry into white, black, and mulatto categories. In 1930 and 1940, census takers were instructed to categorize individuals with white and American Indian ancestry as "Indians," and those of African and American Indian ancestry as "negroes," unless the Indian ancestry predominated. The 2000 U.S. Census reflects renewed expansion of racial options, including five racial categories (American Indian or Alaskan Native, Asian or Pacific Islander, Black, White, and Some Other Race) and two ethnic categories (Hispanic or Latino, and Not Hispanic or Latino) (Daniels and Schulz 2006, 91–92; U.S. Census Bureau 2008). This brief accounting of racial categories in the U.S. reminds us that our understanding of race is less than stable.

Analogously, the historically contingent character of class categories highlights their changing socially and politically constructed nature. To begin with, some definitions of class look only at numerical measures such as wealth or income. Others take into account qualitative factors, such as education, culture, and social status. There is no consensus on which of these variables is essential and which are common. It is also disputed whether sharp lines between classes can be drawn. Sociologist Dennis Gilbert acknowledges that "the class structure . . . does not exactly match the distribution of household income" with "the mismatch [being] greatest in the middle" (Gilbert 1998, 92). As social classes commonly overlap, it is not possible to define exact class boundaries. According to Leonard Beeghley (2004), a household income of roughly $95,000 would be typical for a dual-earner middle-class household whereas $60,000 would be typical for a dual-earner working-class household and $18,000 typical for an impoverished household. Sociologists Joseph Hickey and William Thompson (2007) see common incomes for the upper class as those exceeding $500,000 with upper middle class incomes ranging from the high five figures to most commonly in excess of $100,000. They claim that the lower middle class ranges from $35,000 to $75,000, $16,000 to $30,000 for the working class, and less than $16,000 for the lower class. In 2011, an income of $22,350 or less qualifies a family of four as below the poverty line in forty-eight states and Washington, D.C. (U.S. Census Bureau 2011). The point is that our understanding of class is a changing concept.

A second concern has to do with the problem of stereotyping. Race-based and class-based thinking in nosology and nosography can demonize the carrier and/or group and draw attention away from institutional and social conditions that produce health disparities. Let's consider race-based thinking. It has been typical in medicine to use the term "race" to denote a biological basis for difference between groups of humans (Ossorio 2004). Such groups of individuals are typically labeled as white, black, American Indian, and Asian Pacific Islander (Heron 2010, 12). In medicine, such racial labels are often used in the context of discussing what clinical conditions uniquely affect members of certain populations. It is documented in the genetic literature that cystic fibrosis is expressed in those of Northern European descent, Tays-Sachs in those of Ashkenazi Jewish descent, and sickle cell in those of African descent. Although it is the case that certain clinical conditions tend to express themselves in certain populations, geneticists agree that much further work needs to be done in order to understand the biological bases of such population-based clinical conditions. Further, claims about statistical frequency can lead to stereotyping. By locating the cause of health disparities within the genes—or haplotypes—of racialized groups, geneticists suggest that there is something innately pathologic about that group, thus reinforcing physical inferiority (Daniels and Schulz 2006, 115; also see Gould 1981; Fugh-Berman 2005). Failure to make explicit connections between biological and behavioral factors and race reinforces racial inequalities by playing on racial fears to exacerbate divisions between groups. Shah (2001) describes the explicit construction of the high risk of communicable diseases present among the Chinese immigrants living in cramped, substandard housing in San Francisco, California. Such communicable diseases were constructed as "pestilence" that posed a danger to the "white public" (Shah 2001, 251). They were attributed to the Chinese immigrants themselves, as opposed to the substandard housing in which they were placed (Daniels and Schulz 2006, 99). By locating race in the person or group and not the environment, mistaken biological claims are made and stereotypes are formed that in the end can harm groups of patients.

Analogously, class-based thinking in nosology and nosography can stereotype groups and draw attention away from institutional and social conditions that produce gender-specific disease conditions. It is not unusual in public health discussions to encounter the claim that poverty correlates with disease. Of course, we are reminded that what constitutes "lower class" and "poverty" is not that simple. By locating the cause of health disparities in class or economic status, clinicians suggest that there is something pathologic about that group, thus reinforcing physical inferiority. Failure to make explicit connections between biological and behavioral factors and economic status reinforces class inequalities by playing on class fears to exacerbate divisions between groups. Recently, there has been much discussion about the role of diet in health. Putting aside that our notion of "good" diet has changed over time, typically a "good" diet consisting of fresh products is expensive and sometimes not easily available to those with limited means. Poor Americans are more likely to consume lower quality, processed foods, which is usually less expensive to purchase and more readily available through government-run programs

(Scott 2005). Here, income plays a significant impact on health as those with higher incomes have better access to healthy nutrition and health care facilities. By locating class in a person or group as opposed to the institutional structure of resource allocation, mistaken biological claims are made and stereotypes are formed and perpetuated about the person or group and his or her or their health status.

A third concern has to do with the problem of unresolved tensions between race-based and race-neutral, and class-based and class-neutral, accounts of disease manifestation and treatment. We'll begin with the first tension, one that law professor Patricia King calls "a dilemma of difference" (1992). For King, "[r]ecognizing and taking account of racial differences that have historically been utilized to burden and exploit African Americans pose a dilemma" (King 1992, 36). On the one hand, "in circumstances where the goal of a scientific study is to benefit a stigmatized group or person, such well-intentioned efforts may nevertheless cause harm. If the racial difference is ignored and all groups or persons are treated similarly, unintended harm may result from the failure to recognize racially correlated factors" (King 1992, 36). On the other hand, "if differences among groups or persons are recognized and attempts are made to respond to past injustices or special burdens, the effort is likely to reinforce existing negative stereotypes that contributed to the emphasis on racial differences in the first place" (King 1992, 36). For King, this dilemma is particularly worrisome in medicine. "Because medicine is pragmatic, it will recognize racial differences if doing so will promote health goals. As a consequence, potential harms that might result from attention to racial differences tend to be overlooked, minimized, or viewed as problems beyond the purview of medicine" (King 1992, 37). The challenge in gender-specific medicine becomes navigating between the extreme views that "race is destiny" and "race is irrelevant" in disease expression.

Analogously, a "dilemma of difference" arises with the use of class appeal in medicine. How can medicine begin to address differences in disease expression among classes while preventing against stereotypes and unforeseen consequences that harm patients? If class difference is ignored and all persons and groups are treated similarly, unintended harm may result from the failure to recognize the effects of socio-economic status on health. Conversely, if class difference among persons or groups is recognized, the effect is likely to reinforce existing stereotypes that contributed to the emphasis on class differences in the first place. In medicine, the tension particularly emerges in discussions about access to health care. Given that access to health care can affect who and how one expresses disease, the topic is relevant in this discussion. Those who have difficulty in accessing health care are typically the uninsured. Because the uninsured are often unemployed, they are often poor—or considered lazy in a culture in which access to health care is typically granted by employment. And if the uninsured do seek health care, they are often pushed further into poverty because of the cost of health care services. How can gender-specific practitioners address difference in disease expression among members of particular classes while preventing against stereotypes?

From an integrative standpoint, then, gender-specific medicine will need to be careful in the use of the categories of race/ethnicity and class/socio-economic status because of the ambiguities of the terms, the potential for stereotyping patients, and the challenge of using concepts that one wishes to criticize. It does not follow that such categories of identity and difference ought to be used in analyses of disease expression and treatment. To deny them is to return to a neutral way of approaching disease, and we have already learned about the problems associated with this type of thinking. The message is to proceed carefully with a healthy sense of skepticism about how the terms are defined and to encourage intersectional research on matters concerning gender-specific disease.

SUMMARY

An integrative approach to gender-specific disease seeks a relational, as opposed to an atomistic ontological, understanding of gender-specific disease. It seeks to challenge objectivist, reductionist, positivist, and determinist tendencies in such an understanding. It emphasizes the interdependent and mutually constitutive roles that description and prescription play in framing gender-specific disease within its medical contexts. It emphasizes that gender (and sex) status is one of many factors that influence diseases status. An integrative approach to gender-specific disease leads us to rethink how we understand gender, disease, and their relation.

6 Rethinking Gender-Specific Disease Nomenclature and Taxonomies

TERMINOLOGY AND CLASSIFICATIONS

This chapter considers some of the more practical implications of approaching gender-specific disease integratively. It offers a rethinking of taken-for-granted nomenclature and taxonomy in gender-specific medicine. Drawing from Natalie Stoljar (1995), Alice Dreger (2004), and Eric Juengst (1995), this chapter revisits the language of gender, sex, disease, and disease causation and suggests a rethinking of some of the nomenclature and taxonomies used in gender-specific medicine. It advocates for a rejection of terminology that suggests that gender and sex are static and binomial expressions of nurture and nature (respectively), that disease is a thing out there to be discovered, and that diagnostic terminology promises certainty. It calls for a revision in the language of gender and sex that emphasizes that gender and sex are interrelating continuums involving nature and nurture, disease that emphasizes its multi-factorial character, and diagnostic accounts of causality that acknowledge uncertainty.

GENDER AND SEX

An integrative approach leads us to rethink the nomenclature of gender and sex. As we have learned, as much as we may wish to reduce sex to XX and XY chromosomes, and gender to the social construction of sex, we cannot. Sex is more than chromosomes, and gender more than social forces. The genotype of XX does not equate with the full meaning of what it means to be "female," and the phenotype of "menstruating" does not equate with the full meaning of what it means to be "woman." Further, causal relations among "sex chromosome," clinical phenotype, and gender identity is complex. There is not a direct or simple linear causal relation between each dimension of analysis and it is not possible to arrive at one without the other. Still further, as we have learned, sex and gender are not so separate and distinct. Genetic science has taught us that nature (e.g., biology) and nurture (e.g., the environment) operate in tandem to produce and sustain life. (The genotype of) sex and (the phenotype of) gender are not separate phenomena. Clinicians are unable to study sex outside the boundaries of gender, and gender outside the boundaries of sex. Gender and sex are inter-dependent and mutually constitutive. As humans, we live our bodies, and our bodies are seen through the lenses of our experiences. Given the conclusions of earlier chapters, the suggestion is to begin thinking about gender (and sex) in gender-specific disease in different ways than is represented in the gender-specific medical literature.

Here we might begin with a suggestion made by feminist philosopher Natalie Stoljar. In addressing how to support a category of "woman" without reifying it, Stoljar (1995) suggests focusing on what she calls the resemblance relation held between women of a particular type. She relies on philosopher H.H. Price's resemblance nominalism whereby X is a member of some type F only if X resembles sufficiently some paradigm or exemplar of F (Price 1953, 20). The view here recognizes that we in part discover and in part create experiences of natural phenomena by organizing observations in terms of patterns that in turn function as categories of reference and action (see as well Chapter 2). For Stoljar, woman is a cluster concept and our attribution of womanhood picks out "different arrangements of features in different individuals" (Stoljar 2000, 27). More specifically, they pick out features representing (a) biological ones, such as organs, specified levels of hormones, chromosomes; (b) phenomenological or experiential ones, such as breast development, menstruation, feminine sexual experience, childbirth; (c) select roles, such as wearing typical feminine clothing, undertaking work typical of women; and (d) gender self-attribution, such as "calling oneself a woman, being called a woman" (Stoljar 1995, 283–84).

Stoljar's account of gender and sex acknowledges what we have already concluded in the foregoing analysis, that our concepts of gender and sex are never "pure"; they are embedded within scientific language and interpretations of meaning and practice that humans bring to their experience of a biological/sociological/psychological phenomenon. Still further the meaning of gender and sex interrelate. Chromosomes are understood through the lens of embodied beings, and embodied beings through select biological frameworks. Given the range of gender and sexual expression that are evident, we arrive at an understanding of the sex/gender dyad in terms of a continuum. Consider the suggested schema below based on Stoljar's analysis of "woman":

Sex/Gender Types

features/type	1	2	3	4	5	6	7	8	9	10	11	12	13	14
(a) biology	f	f	f	f	f	f	f	m	m	m	m	m	m	m
(b) experience	f	m	f	f	m	f	m	m	f	m	m	f	m	f
(c) roles	F	F	M	F	M	M	M	M	M	F	M	F	F	F
(d) self-attribution	F	F	F	M	F	M	M	M	M	M	F	M	F	F

Key: (what is traditionally seen as)
f = female; m = male; F = feminine; M = masculine

Figure 6.1   Classifying sex/gender types.

The schema above illustrates how our understanding of sex and gender interrelate to create categories of analysis that we experience. There are those who fit into type 1 (the traditionally- speaking female and feminine) and type 8 (the traditionally-speaking male and masculine). There are those who fit into other types of sex/gender as well.

Consider a case of type 13. Spanish Olympian hurdler Maria Patiño has XY chromosomes, male genitalia, is considered by others to be a woman, and considers herself a woman. In the 1980s, Patiño successfully fought in court to be recognized as a female athlete, arguing that her chromosomes alone were not sufficient for her sexual identity in sports (Fausto-Sterling 2000b, 1–3). In a more recent case, and as illustration of type 6, "the pregnant man" Thomas Beatie has XX chromosomes, female genitalia, is considered by his wife to be a man, and considers himself a man. He successfully fought in an Oregon court to be recognized as a male, arguing that the results of his psychological testing indicated that he considers himself a man. He went on to have his breasts surgically removed and bore his first child in June 2008. A second child was born on June 10, 2009 ("Pregnant man" 2009; see also the case of Chaz Bono [2011]).

In addition, there will be those (type 4) who see themselves as a man, but who have XX chromosomes and female genitalia, and who others call a "she." There will be those (type 11) who consider themselves a woman, with XY chromosomes and male genitalia, and who others call a "he." There will be those (type 3) who others call a "he," but who have XX chromosomes and female genitalia, and who see themselves as a "she." There will be those (type 10) who others call a "she," but who have XY chromosomes and male genitalia, and who see themselves as a "he." This type of approach to talking about sex and gender challenges a taken-for-granted assumption in contemporary medicine, namely, that the determination of sex starts with chromosomal analysis and leads to behavioral ones and the determination of gender. It illustrates instead how a combination of incongruous biological, experience-based, and identity-based factors come together in order to demarcate how we understand types of sex and gender.

The point here is to encourage reevaluation of the taxonomies and nomenclature of sex and gender. As Lorber says, "[c]ategories [of sex and gender] could be broken up and people regrouped differently into new categories for comparison. This process of discovering categories from similarities and differences in people's behavior or responses can be more meaningful . . . than discovering similarities and differences between "females" and "males" or "women" and "men" because the social construction of the conventional sex and gender categories already assumes differences between them and similarities among them" (Lorber 1995, 42). Lorber's point is that because the categories we embrace already assume a structure of reality, we may not be able to rethink our assumptions and claims without changing the categories or lenses themselves (also see Foucault 1978; Klausner 2005).

A reconception of sex and gender is admittedly a radical move in medicine (and culture) and will involve revolutionary changes in how and what medicine thinks about gender and sex. We can learn something about the challenge that comes with rethinking nomenclature and taxonomies in gender-specific medicine from who have taken on analogous tasks. Earlier we considered changes in how medicine has begun to talk about "intersex" types. These changes came about in response to concerns about the stereotypes that have been fostered by the language of "hermaphrodite" in medicine. In recommending new ways to talk and think about "intersex" types, Dreger et al. (2005) suggest that a replacement taxonomic system:

> *should* enhance, not complicate, the use of medical informatics in research and clinical practice;
> *should* recognize that diagnosis and taxonomy inform, but do not determine, gender assignment and/or gender identity ([and] thus, should avoid the words "male" and "female");
> should *not* include the words 'hermaphrodite', 'hermaphroditism', 'sex reversal' , or other easily misunderstood terms;
> *should* label the condition rather than the person;
> should *not* confuse physicians and patients;
> *should* make clear that diagnosis does not simply dictate therapy (Dreger et al. 2005, 733).

In response to these types of suggestions, an interdisciplinary team of health care practitioners, patients, and interested parties arrived at a recommendation to develop clinical language for intersex types that is carefully descriptive and reflective of genetic etiology and accommodates phenotypical variations (Hughes et al. 2006).

Applied to our discussion of gender-specific disease, in rethinking its language, gender-specific medicine will want to (1) use language that reflects proper medical informatics in gender-specific research and clinical practice, (2) be cautious about asserting that gender-specific diagnoses determine gender-assignments, (3) avoid terms that are misleading or misunderstood,

(4) focus on clinical conditions rather than the assumed gender assignment of the person, (5) use language that is clear to both clinicians and patients, and (6) recognize that diagnosis should not dictate therapy. What definitions and diagnostic labels of gender-specific disease are developed will require an interdisciplinary discussion involving health care practitioners, patients, and interested parties in order to ensure that the criteria above are met and problematic stereotypes and claims are avoided.

One suggestion is to move away from the language of "woman" and "man," and "female" and "male," in the gender-specific disease literature. As indicated in earlier discussions, there is good support in gender-specific medicine for using the language of underlying genetic and endocrine factors that lead to gender-specific expressions that bring patients to the attention of health care professionals. Although there is an advantage in calling for as much precision as possible offered by the genetic etiology of gender-specific disease conditions, caution is encouraged. As we have learned in the previous chapters, we will mislead ourselves if we think that genetic explanations will solve all of the challenges in developing accounts of gender-specific disease conditions. This is because genetic explanations involve their own objectivist, reductionist, positivist, and determinist assumptions and claims. Instead, combining phenotypical analysis with karyotype, gonadal histology, and etiology may be the direction to proceed in gender-specific medicine in order to arrive at new language for gender and sex. But again, this is a discussion for a much larger group of thinkers, one involving gender-specific practitioners as well as patients and representatives of gender advocacy groups in order to arrive at clinical language that will be scientifically accurate, practically useful, and socially and morally acceptable.

DISEASE

An integrative approach leads us to rethink the taxonomies and nomenclature of disease as well. As the International Classification of Disease (ICD) recognizes, classifications of disease are no longer simply based on signs and symptoms, as was the case when seventeenth-century Thomas Sydenham practiced medicine. Although the isolation of signs and symptoms provides a basis for making repeated observations in the clinic and for recommending treatments that target symptoms, this type of approach to disease is by itself insufficient to determine the wide range of disease conditions experienced by patients. Etiological accounts of disease allow the isolation of direct and indirect causes of conditions that lead to biological dysfunction and the associated pain and suffering reported by patients. They guide the development of preventive and curative treatments and seek to change the course of the disease. But this too by itself has its limits. Disease involves a cluster of ways to explain clinical events, as we see in the International Classification of Disease taxonomy that defines disease in terms of:

1. *symptomatology—manifestations*: known pattern of signs, symptoms and related findings
2. *etiology*: an underlying explanatory mechanism
3. *course and outcome*: a distinct pattern of development over time
4. *treatment response*: a known pattern of response to interventions
5. *linkage to genetic factors*: e.g., genotypes, patterns of gene expression
6. *linkage to interacting environmental factors* (Production of ICD-11: The Revision Process 2007)

In the case of gender-specific disease, one can expect that there will be diseases defined by symptoms (e.g., rheumatoid arthritis), etiology (e.g., AIDS), course and outcome (e.g., arterial hypertension), response to treatment (e.g., hypothyroidism), genetics (e.g., X-linked conditions), and environmental factors (e.g., tobacco-related lung cancer). In the end, disease is a multi-factorial concept which guides a host of ways to treat patients.

Given this, medicine might further consider that "linkage to gender-specific factors" might serve a fruitful category in the upcoming decades in light of new knowledge emerging in gender-specific medicine. Such a category serves to highlight the interacting role played by etiological and environmental factors in disease expression such that it is difficult to single out one type of factor as more important than another. Such a multi-factorial account of disease is reflective of what we understand as disease—as a host of factors involving physiological processes and environmental influences coming together in such a way to lead to conditions that we call a "disease."

Put another way, disease can at best be understood in terms of a clinical model that guides the development of clinical recipes (Cutter 2003). Clinical models provide a way to view disease in terms of numerous intervening variables where certain variables are singled out as more important than others depending on the perspective brought to the clinical event. Immunologists will focus on immunological events, geneticists on genetic events, and gender-specific practitioners on gender-specific factors. The possibility of dealing effectively and efficiently with what comes into the clinic provides clinical models a practical advantage in contemporary medicine. Clinical recipes single out those means that are more effectively and efficiently manipulated for purposes of achieving the goal of addressing the biological dysfunction and/or pain and suffering associated with it.

A multi-factorial approach to disease is in keeping with an integrative approach to disease supported in the prior analysis. Disease is integrative, or a function of numerous and overlapping variables that lead to biological dysfunction experienced by patients. Understanding disease in terms of a multi-factorial model of biological dysfunction experienced by patients within particular contexts is also in keeping with the state of medicine today. Medicine today is composed of multiple and overlapping departments and disciplines, a legacy that health care professionals carry with them as they pursue their specialties and in turn join various health care teams and discussions in medicine. This is not to suggest that the integration of medicine is as it should be. As we have seen, integrative clinicians (recall Weil and Northrup) say too often specialists fail to consider the interrelation among variables (e.g., physiological or anatomical dysfunction, family history, lifestyle habits, diet, environmental influences) that contribute to disease. An integrative approach to disease challenges the taken-for-granted view of disease as a thing out there to be discovered and highlights its multi-factorial character.

GENDER-SPECIFIC DISEASE CAUSATION

An integrative approach leads us to rethink the nomenclature of disease causation within the context of clinical diagnostics. As we have learned, disease causation in medicine can be understood in terms of necessary, sufficient, contributory, and manipulative relations. Although medicine may aspire to uncover necessary and sufficient causal relations between gender and disease, it is usually working with contributory and manipulatory ones. As Gøtzsche says, "when it is stated that the aetiology is known it usually only means that one of the many aetiological factors has been isolated, and when it is stated that the pathogenesis is known, it usually only means that a few links in the chain of events leading to the observed clinical picture have been discovered" (Gøtzsche 2007, 56). Contributory and manipulatory causal relations focus on the links in the causal chain leading to disease, and on what can be manipulated in order to change the conditions of the disease.

This recognition of the different levels of certainty provided by causal claims in medicine is an opportunity to reflect on diagnostic language in gender-specific medicine. One can envision, as philosopher Eric Juengst (1995, 2004) has in the context of genetic medicine, that degrees of certainty can be assigned to different aspects and procedures in medical testing akin to the differentiation we commonly accept in the legal context: from probable cause and circumstantial evidence to evidence or eye-witness testimony that is beyond a shadow of a doubt. These degrees of certainty, or rather uncertainty, range from diagnostic, prognostic, and prophylactic to probabilistic assessments, depending on what is known and how it is known. Adopting Juengst's language to our discussion of gender-specific disease, we arrive at the following senses of diagnosis of medical testing for gender-specific disease:

(1) "Diagnostic" is reserved for gender-specific factors that can be used to confirm the diagnosis of an active gender-specific disease (e.g., BRCA).

(2) "Prognostic" or "presymptomatic" is reserved for gender-specific factors that are capable of being used to forecast the emergence of a gender-specific disease with a large degree of certainty (e.g., the use of mutation analysis to diagnose fragile-X syndrome in developmentally delayed males).

(3) "Prophylactic" is reserved for gender-specific factors that confer gender-specific vulnerability to a disease and for which "external" interventions may be offered (e.g., alpha-1-antitripsin deficiency—in the absence of tobacco smoke, it does no harm but in those who smoke, it represents a serious liability, and in females because of their heightened vulnerability to tobacco toxins, it represent even more of a liability).

(4) "Probabilistic" is reserved for a less determined category of gender-specific risk assessment which alerts patients that they are statistically at a higher risk than the population for a particular health problem (e.g., osteoporosis).

These senses of gender-specific testing serve to caution against simplistic interpretations of clinical causation and the predictive power of clinical tests in the context of talking about gender-specific disease.

It is important to recognize that uncertainty is not just a result of not having enough information in a world of limited research. It would be prudent to recognize the underlying forces encouraging us not to know. This is especially important in medicine because of its power to change lives. Feminist philosopher Nancy Tuana (2006) reminds us that an understanding of knowledge must be accompanied by an understanding of the practices that account for *not* knowing. Here, according to Tuana, the notion of ignorance is complex and involves the ways in which we do not care about knowing (e.g., male contraceptives), we don't know what we don't know (e.g., the unique physiology of the female), we don't know because others do not want us to know (e.g., dangerous side effects of oral contraceptives), and we do not know because we refuse to know (e.g., incest in the home). In the case of gender-specific disease, one might think of the ways in which we do not care about knowing (e.g., the unique health challenges of members of the lesbian, gay, transgender, and bisexual communities), we don't know what we do not know (e.g., gender differences in many diseases), we do not know because others do not want us to know (e.g., the extent to which medical knowledge is uncertain), and we do not know because we refuse to know (e.g., how the language of "gender" and "sex" need revision). We cannot begin to appreciate what we know until we recognize what we do not know and why. In other words, epistemologies of knowledge go hand-in-hand with epistemologies of ignorance. In the case of gender-specific medicine, this insight carries particular urgency because of the recent interest in gender-specific medicine and the challenge that comes with addressing gender in medicine.

CONCEPTS OF GENDER-SPECIFIC DISEASE

One of the insights we can draw from an integrative approach to gender-specific disease is that it will be more accurate to talk about "concepts," as opposed to a "concept," of gender-specific disease. Drawing from philosopher David Magnus (2004) who addresses concepts of disease in genetic medicine, consider how we arrive at concepts of disease in gender-specific medicine. In the case of determining the necessary and sufficient cause of gender-specific disease, what counts as disease depends on the ability to determine the direct cause, which in the case of gender-specific disease are the gender-specific factors that function as important variables of disease. This is in keeping with a naturalist view of disease, the view that a disease is a real entity and independent of factors outside the disease (recall Boorse 1975, 1977). Determining the direct cause has the advantage of fitting the clinical ideal of finding the "magic bullet" for a particular disease condition, but in medicine, as we have already discussed, this ideal is often not achievable. Further, in the case of gender-specific disease, the ideal of direct cause is particularly challenging in light of the difficulty of determining how gender-specific factors cause disease. Thus, other approaches to gender-specific disease causation are needed.

In the case of determining the contributory cause of gender-specific disease, what counts as disease depends on the population it is a part of. It depends on large-scale data about what factors in a gendered population typically contribute to particular disease outcomes. It depends on population-based statistical analysis of the gender-specific factors that lead to disease. This is in keeping with a public health view of disease, and whereas it is helpful for determining the epidemiology of disease, it may be less helpful in the clinic, which tends to focus on an individual patient. Knowing that X% of the population expresses Y disease may be of epidemiological interest, but the opportunity to know whether *I* have a disease is usually what brings me into the clinic. This will be no different in gender-specific medicine.

In the case of the manipulability account of causation, what counts as gender-specific disease depends on the ability to manipulate it. This in turn depends on technological advances. Current medicine relies heavily on technological advances and it is no wonder why the number of nosologies and nosographies has rapidly grown in the latter part of the twentieth century during a time when medical technology has increasingly developed. A manipulability account of gender-specific disease is in keeping with the view that gender and disease are prescriptive notions. Determining cause based on what can be manipulated has the distinct advantage that it works. The course of gender-specific disease can be changed even when the cause of the disease cannot be known. The disadvantage of a manipulatory account of causation is that diseases that cannot be manipulated or treated cannot be fully understood.

Given the inability to provide any single definitive account of the concept of gender-specific disease, it follows that there are "concepts," as opposed to a "concept," of gender-specific disease. There are varying accounts of gender, ranging from a biological phenomenon (akin to sex) to a dimension of analysis that reflects social and psychological roles humans assume. It entails varying accounts of disease, ranging from a biological entity to a warrant for treatment. It entails varying accounts of disease causation, ranging from an account of the "direct" causal relation between gender-specific factors and disease to an "indirect" account to an account of what can be manipulated.

Yet, it does not follow that anything goes in gender-specific disease classification. There may be clinical categories that may not be appropriate candidates for gender-specific disease status because of the wide-spread implications of overuse, stigmatization, and mistreatment. Here one is reminded of the history of the clinical classification of homosexuality. The clinical concept of homosexuality developed from an instance of "sociopathic personality disturbance" in the first Diagnostic and Statistical Manual of the American Psychiatric Association (DSM-I) (APA 1952, 38–39) to a "personality disorder" in DSM-II (APA 1968, 44, taxon 302.0). Under pressure to change, the American Psychiatric Association reclassified the clinical concept of homosexuality as an instance of "psychosocial dysfunction" in DSM-III (APA 1980, 281, taxon 302.00) under the taxon "ego-dystonic homosexuality" and then as an instance in DSM-III-R (APA 1987, 296, taxon 302.90) of "sexual dysfunction" under the obscure taxon "sexual disorder not otherwise specified," in a way that includes heterosexuals' "persistent and marked distress about their sexual orientation." In DSM-IV (APA 1994, 538, taxon 302.9) and DSM-IV-R (APA 2000), homosexuality remains under the same rubric as in DSM-III-R. Today, homosexuality (as well as other classifications of sexuality) is seen to be a mental disorder only if the individual has a persistent concern to change sexual orientation. The shift in the medicalization of homosexuality provides insight into how changes in ideas of sexuality, the notion of perversion, and views regarding the proper bounds of disease language influence how disease is classified.

SUMMARY

An integrative approach to gender-specific disease leads us to rethink the use of nomenclature and taxonomies in gender-specific medicine. Gender-specific medicine has the unique opportunity to reconsider its use of gender, sex, disease, and the diagnostic language used to convey disease causation. Based on the reflections here, it is more accurate to represent gender and sex as intersecting continuums, disease as a multi-factorial expression of disvalued biological dysfunction, and disease causation as less than certain. What nomenclature and taxonomies are adopted and employed will be determined through a larger discussion than what is found here. Perhaps this discussion serves as an impetus to begin such a discussion.

7 Toward an Integrative Bioethics

KNOWING AND ETHICALLY VALUING

To see a clinical phenomenon as a gender-specific disease is to observe a level of gender-specific biological dysfunction or expect there to be one if the clinical course continues. It is to judge a clinical phenomenon as failing to achieve an expected state. This may be a failure to reach an ideal level of freedom from pain or suffering. It may involve a failure to achieve a realization of human form or grace or a failure to attain what is an expected span of life. These genres of judgment characterize a clinical circumstance as one of suffering, one of pathology, and one of a problem to be solved. Such judgments turn on a variety of forces including background commitments regarding the rules of evidence and inference in medicine that reflect professional, consumer, and societal goals. They turn as well on ethical or moral considerations concerning what ought or ought not to be done in certain situations. This recognition of the normative implications of knowing, and the epistemological implications of ethical valuing, underscores our choices and indicates our responsibilities as individuals who know reality in order to manipulate it, and manipulate it in order to know it. We find ourselves squarely lodged in the ethical challenges and opportunities raised by understanding gender-specific disease.

This and the next chapter present some of the ethical or moral implications of approaching gender-specific disease integratively. This chapter sets the stage for the argument that the methodological approach used in bioethics to assess gender-specific disease descriptions and prescriptions needs to be integrative. It reviews the popular principle-based approach developed by contemporary bioethicists Tom L. Beauchamp and James F. Childress (2009) and shows its limits when it comes to assessing gender-specific disease. With the help of Rosemarie Tong (1997) and other feminist philosophers, the chapter shows the need for a gender-inclusive approach in order to assess bioethical concerns raised by our understanding of gender-specific disease. The next chapter continues the methodological analysis and argues for a gender-inclusive bioethical approach that is integrative. Taken together, this and the next chapter illustrate that our understanding of gender-specific disease carries ethical implications for the bioethical methodologies we use and the practices we follow in gender-specific medicine.

GENDER-NEUTRAL BIOETHICS

Bioethics (Gr. *bio*, "life" + Gr. *ēthikē*, "ethical," or study of standards of conduct) is the study of the ethical or moral implications of biomedical discoveries and practices. It gained notoriety at the end of the twentieth century for its incisive analyses and critiques of practices in medicine. The term "bioethics" was coined by Dr. Van Rensselaer Potter, a research oncologist at the University of Wisconsin in the early 1970s (Jonsen 1998, 27). Potter published an article in 1970 entitled "Bioethics, the Science of Survival" (1970) and, in 1971, followed it with his book *Bioethics: Bridge to the Future*. Potter defined bioethics as "a new discipline that combines biological knowledge with a knowledge of human value systems" (1971, 2). Bioethics has since become influential in western medicine especially as we become increasingly concerned about the role, power, and limits of medicine in our lives and as bioethicists enter into mainstream medical school teaching and research to offer analyses and critiques of medical practices.

One of the most influential approaches in bioethics today is referred to as a "principle-based approach" or "principlism" and employs the language of autonomy, non-maleficence, beneficence, and justice to address ethical transgressions in medicine (Beauchamp and Childress 2009 [first published 1979]). It is by far, and over the years, the most influential text in the field of bioethics. It has shaped the very character of bioethics as well as what constitutes ethical clinical practice, research protocols, and health policies. Let's consider the major principles and how they can guide thinking about the ethicality of framing gender-specific disease.

The "Patient Rights Movement," as it is often called, has successfully argued that patients have a right to receive the care that medicine deems appropriate for their clinical conditions. This view is based on a patient's right to autonomy and instructs each person to acknowledge another's "right to hold views, to make choices, and to take actions based on personal values and beliefs" (Beauchamp and Childress 2009, 103). The principle of autonomy is a moral and legal concept rooted in the thinking of philosopher Immanuel Kant (1985 [1785]) and his position that respect for a person is a necessary condition of the possibility of the moral community. As Kant says, "[a]ct so that you treat humanity, whether in your own person or in that of another always as an end and never as a means only" (Kant 1985 [1785], 47). The principle of autonomy requires the treatment of another as an end, and not as a means. It requires the non-interference of another's attitudes and actions as well as an obligation to build up or maintain another's "capacities for autonomous choice while helping to allay fears and other conditions that destroy or disrupt their autonomous action" (Beauchamp and Childress 2009, 103). Put practically, in medicine, autonomy grounds truth-telling, respect for the privacy of others, protection of confidential information, and the practice of informed consent (Beauchamp and Childress 2009, 104).

The principle of autonomy successfully focuses our attention on the centrality of honoring patient rights in the health care setting. For some (Nozick 1974), autonomy is a side-constraint in the moral life and any restrictions other than minimal protections of autonomy violate autonomy. But there are additional ethical principles that highlight aspects of an ethical clinical encounter that have to do with patient welfare. On the one hand, there is the long-standing ethical mandate in medicine to "do no harm." The principle of non-maleficence "imposes an obligation not to inflict harm on others" (Beauchamp and Childress 2009, 149). It involves intentionally *refraining* from actions that cause harm. The principle of non-maleficence has come to be closely associated with the familiar maxim *Primum non nocere*, "above all [or first] do not harm," a notion rooted in Hippocratic thinking (Hippocrates 1923 [fifth c. B.C.E.], 165). It supports specific moral actions in medicine such as refraining from killing, causing pain or suffering, incapacitating another, causing offense, and depriving another of the goods of life (Beauchamp and Childress 2009, 149–50).

Tied to the ethical mandate to prevent patient harm is another long-standing ethical mandate to promote patient welfare. Whereas the principle of non-maleficence calls for refrain from action, the principle of beneficence "requires taking action by *helping*—preventing harm, removing harm, and promoting good" (Beauchamp and Childress 2009, 151), much in the tradition of John Stuart Mill's (1979 [1861]) ethical mandate to promote the best interest of another. As Mill says, "The creed which accepts as the foundation of morals 'utility' or 'the greatest happiness principle' holds that actions are right in proportion as they tend to promote happiness; wrong as they tend to produce the reverse of happiness" (Mill 1979 [1861], 7). The principle of beneficence supports *general* rules of moral actions such as protecting and defending the rights of others, preventing harm from occurring to others, removing conditions that will cause harm to others, helping persons with disabilities, and rescuing persons in danger (Beauchamp and Childress 2009, 199ff).

The principle of beneficence supports *specific* rules directed at persons such as children, friends, and patients. Beauchamp and Childress argue that a person (X) has a specific obligation of beneficence toward person (Y) if and only if each of the following conditions is satisfied:

1. Y is at risk of significant loss or damage to life or health or some other major interest.
2. X's action is necessary (singly or in concert with others) to prevent this loss or damage.
3. X's action (singly or in concert with each other) has a very high probability of preventing it.
4. X's action would not present very significant risks, costs, or burdens to X.

5. The benefit that Y can be expected to gain outweighs any harms, costs, or burdens that X is likely to incur (Beauchamp and Childress 2009, 202).

In thinking through the requirements of beneficent actions, much turns on what constitutes "significant risks, costs, or burdens," for which informal and formal techniques have been developed. Informal techniques include "expert judgments based on reliable data and analogical reasoning based on precedents" (Beauchamp and Childress 2009, 221). These techniques are typically used in Institutional Review Board (IRB) protocol, where the investigator must state the risks to subjects and probable benefits to both subjects and society and justify how the probable benefits outweigh the risks to the subject. Formal, quantitative techniques involve "the analysis of costs, risks, and benefits" (Beauchamp and Childress 2009, 221). This is a sophisticated body of techniques, much too much to review here, but for purposes of illustration involve cost-effectiveness analysis (CEA, which measures the benefits in non-monetary terms such as years of life, quality-adjusted-life-years or QALYS, and cases of disease), cost-benefit analysis (CBA, which measures both the benefits and costs in monetary terms), and risk-benefit analysis (RBA, which evaluates risks in relation to probable benefits).

Not only are the principles of autonomy, non-maleficence, and beneficence central to a principle-based approach in contemporary bioethics, justice is as well. The principle of justice guides our thinking about what is fair, equitable, and appropriate in light of what is due or owed to persons. Justice is one of the oldest moral principles dating back to the Ancient Greek philosopher Aristotle (384–322 B.C.E.) (1941). As Aristotle said, "the just, then, is the lawful and the fair, the unjust the unlawful and the unfair" (1941, 1129a 34–35). Common to all theories of justice is Aristotle's mandate to treat equals equally, and unequals unequally. "This principle of justice . . . is 'formal' because it identifies no particular situations in which equals are to be treated equally and provides no criteria for determining whether two or more individuals are in fact equals" (Beauchamp and Childress 2009, 242). Although this reading of Aristotle is oversimplified, it emphasizes how our understanding of justice depends on the criteria that are used to evaluate it.

In the principle-based approach, justice is commonly distinguished as distributive, criminal, and rectificatory. Distributive justice "refers to fair, equitable, and appropriate distribution determined by justified norms that structure the terms of social cooperation. Its scope includes policies that allot diverse benefits and burdens such as property, resources, taxation, privileges, and opportunities" (Beauchamp and Childress 2009, 241). Criminal justice addresses the appropriate "infliction of punishment" (2009, 241) as set forth by a body of law. This includes estimates about what kind and degree of punishment is appropriate in certain situations, as well as what might be done to rehabilitate a criminal. Rectificatory justice attends to the fair "compensation [to victims] for transaction problems such as breach of contracts and malpractice" (2009, 241). This includes estimates about what kind and degree of compensation are appropriate in particular situations.

A variety of "material" or "substantive" principles of justice has been proposed and includes distribution according to equal share, need, effort, contribution, merit, and free-market exchanges (Beauchamp and Childress 2009, 243). In some sense, one's material view of justice turns on how one weighs the ethical demands to protect the rights and welfare of the parties involved. The more one holds that rights are to be protected at all costs, the more one will view justice in terms of the following libertarian maxim: "*From each as they choose, to each as they are chosen*" (Nozick 1974, 160, *italics in original*). Here justice does not require any type of equal distribution among equals; it only requires that each person be treated as having forbearance rights, i.e., rights to be left alone (which are admittedly not the focus of Beauchamp and Childress's analysis of justice). Alternatively, the more one holds that welfare is to be protected at all costs, the more one will view justice in terms of the following communitarian maxim: "to each according to individual need or benefit" (ten Have and Keasberry 1992). In the "middle," so to speak, are views regarding restricting either the protection of individual rights or individual and/or societal welfare. For the former, the maxims might be "to each according to what one chooses insofar as individual needs or benefits are met" and the latter "to each according to individual needs or benefits with exceptions made for protecting rights." These are various accounts of justice, ranging in the traditions of classical liberal John Locke (1632–1704) (1980 [1690]), utilitarian John Stuart Mill (1806–1873) (1979 [1861]), and egalitarian John Rawls (1971).

The principle-based approach has fostered a rich discussion about how to order the ethical principles. For Beauchamp and Childress, the human power of judgment determines which principle has priority over the other in a particular situation (2009, 381ff). As they say, "[m]ethod in ethics properly begins with our 'considered judgments,' which are the moral convictions in which we have the highest confidence and believe to have the least bias" (2009, 382). The quality of least bias or minimal distortion is more than "correct" judgment. "It refers to the conditions under which the judgments are formed" (2009, 382). Considered judgments "occur at all levels of generality in moral thinking" (2009, 382), from particular ones through formal and abstract conditions on moral conceptions. Drawing from philosopher John Rawls (1971) and his account of reflective equilibrium, Beauchamp and Childress instruct that "[w]henever some feature in a moral theory that we hold conflicts with one or more of our considered judgments . . . we must modify one or the other to achieve equilibrium" (2009, 382).

There is no doubt that the principle-based approach in bioethics has assisted us in addressing some of the ethical implications of gendering disease. The recognition of autonomy benefited and continues to benefit women patients and research subjects in medicine. It has demanded the treatment of a woman as an end and not means and protected a woman's capacity for autonomous decision-making. It has secured a zone of privacy for women protecting them in their most personal health-related decisions, and especially reproductive ones (see, e.g., *Griswold v. Connecticut* 1965; *Roe v. Wade* 1973). In the context of gender-specific medicine, a principle-based approach would expect a similar commitment to protecting patient autonomy. In developing accounts of gender-specific disease, gender-specific medicine will need to ensure accurate information about the gender-specific factors that bring diseases about in order to make possible patient consent and to ensure beneficial consequences.

The imperative to minimize harms and maximize benefits advantaged and continues to advantage women in clinical practice and research by emphasizing the need for less harmful and more beneficial health care for women. This imperative has been grounds for successful campaigns for more research on medical conditions that affect women (Women's Health Initiative 2007) and a serious reevaluation of taken-for-granted medical procedures that particularly affect women, such as radical mastectomies, caesarian section, hormone replacement therapy, etc. As already has been discussed, almost two-thirds of the diseases and their treatments that affect both females and males have been studied exclusively in men (DeLorey 2007). The situation was deemed so serious that federal regulations were revised to require the participation of females in government-funded research protocols (see Chapter 1). Increased information and more accurate diagnostics and treatments for gender-specific medical conditions have benefited women by reducing patient suffering, helping patients to return to a desired level of function, and preventing the onset of debilitating conditions. Such goals reflect a moral commitment to prevent harms to women, to remove harms from women, and to promote their welfare.

The call for justice in health care has also served women well. It has brought to our attention the moral imperative that "no persons should receive social benefits on the basis of undeserved advantageous properties (because no persons are responsible for having these properties) and that no persons should be denied social benefits on the basis of undeserved disadvantageous properties (because they also are not responsible for these properties)" (Beauchamp and Childress 2009, 248). Properties, such as gender, race, ethnicity, IQ, national origin, and social status, are not chosen by individuals and thus do not provide grounds for morally accepted discrimination (Beauchamp and Childress 2009, 248–49). The call for justice in health care has brought to attention disparities in women's health care and research that have arisen from inadequate diagnostics and treatments for their health care problems (Council on Ethical and Judicial Affairs 1991;

Institute of Medicine 2001a). This recognition has fueled greater efforts to advance knowledge about gender-specific diseases with hopes that there can be more attention to gender-specific research and practice.

This may be a good start in helping craft a reaction to the ethical challenge of gendering disease. It focuses on some of the concerns we have about the use and misuse of gender-specific diagnostics and treatments. Violations of rights, the undermining of welfare, and unjust misappropriations of resources are serious and problematic ethical implications of misframing, misusing, and ignoring the need for gender-specific diagnostics and interventions. But in light of the epistemological analysis that has taken place in early chapters, an ethical analysis of the moral implications of framing gender-specific disease has only begun. As we will see, it will entail an evaluation of the bioethical approach itself that we use to assess gender-specific matters. When such an assessment takes place, one finds that the very method popularly used in contemporary bioethics is limited in helping us uncover some of the ethical problems that can occur in framing gender-specific disease.

GENDER-INCLUSIVE BIOETHICS

Although its role in forging advancements in women's lives is unquestioned, the principle-based approach can be criticized for offering in the end "little attention to gender-specific disparities in health care research and therapy and the effects of racial and class differences on quality of care" (Donchin 2009). Beauchamp and Childress's best-selling principle-based approach in bioethics contains no more than eight references to gender, and when it does, the entries are brief, rehearsing the (singular) tradition of "care ethics" (2009, 35–38) and popular medico-legal cases such as the *Auto Workers v. Johnson Controls, Inc.* (1991), which argues that the prohibition of women of child-bearing age from working in hazardous workplaces is illegal on grounds that it discriminates based on gender (2009, 244). Lack of attention to how gender is understood in such contexts results in a lack of appreciation of the relational networks that inform patient decision-making, welfare, and access to clinical services. This can lead in turn to inadequate ethical analyses of how to understand gender-specific disease.

Feminists from a variety of disciplines, including philosophy, sociology, and women's studies, have spent much time addressing how sex, gender, and other categories of analyses are bound up with power relations across public and private spheres. They have given special attention to the role of gender in reproductive services, birthing practices, breast health, hormone use, research involving women, and AIDS, to name a few. They have championed changes in medicine that have led to new policies and laws. Feminist work has been both theoretical and practical in bringing about awareness of the need to address the role of gender in medicine (Donchin 2009). What follows draws from some of the major contributions in thinking through what has come to be known as "feminist bioethics" in order to illustrate the ethical implications of framing gender-specific disease. My intention is to provide an overview of feminist contributions in bioethics (as opposed to any detailed analysis) and show the relevancy of some of the thinking found in this body of thought for reflecting upon how to engage in bioethical thinking about gendering disease. It is the application (to the case of gendering disease), and not the theory, that marks what follows as unique.

It is first helpful to recognize that feminist approaches to a gender-inclusive bioethics are not monolithic. They rather entail a variety of methods and concerns, including what feminist bioethicist Rosemarie Tong (1997) calls "care ethics" and "power ethics." Care ethics (Tong 1997) came on the scene in bioethics in the early 1980s and focuses attention on the psychological aspects of moral decision-making, with an emphasis on how persons of differing genders make decisions (Manning 1992; Noddings 1984). Psychologist Carol Gilligan (1982) questioned her mentor Lawrence Kohlberg's (1984) earlier studies that concluded that women are "less developed" in their moral reasoning skills than men because they did not apply moral principles as universally as men did. Men, Kohlberg reports, tend to focus on a moral dilemma with the aim of deciding which abstract rule applies that may solve the case. In her studies, Gilligan found that when women are presented with cases of moral conflicts, they focus on the details of the people involved in the situation and their personal relationships. In attempting to resolve the dilemma, women look for compromises and points of agreement, are flexible in their demands, and often take novel approaches to find resolutions. Care ethics rejects the view that abstract principles can capture that which is relevant in making moral decisions. Some (e.g., Nel Noddings 1984) favor dispensing with principles entirely and reconstituting bioethics through narrative case-specific interpretation. Others (e.g., Lynn Hankinson Nelson 2001) argue that narratives should be one of the tools in the bioethicist's methodological toolbox. A focus on care and how different decisions affect the relations of the parties involved in the medical setting is seen to be an appropriate fit.

Power ethics (Tong 1997) also rejects the traditional notion that ethics can be represented by a set of abstract principles and that the morality of actions and policies can be assessed by reference to them. For feminist philosopher Alison Jaggar, power-focused approaches begin "from the conviction that the subordination of women is morally wrong and that the moral experience of women is as worthy of respect as those of men" (1992, 361). On this view, ethics is part of an ongoing effort to uncover and eliminate sources of social inequality or oppression. Part of rooting out the sources is looking at the nature of ethics itself. Traditionally, the discipline of ethics has been in many ways itself a product of the privileged male's domination over women. An emphasis on individual rights, for instance, shows preference toward men who were rights holders, property owners, and rational agents well before women. An emphasis on welfare shows preference toward those in society, in this case men, whose interests were seen to be worthy of promotion. An emphasis on justice (in the traditional sense) focuses on abstract generalizations about moral agents and attends to who deserves what based on such generalizations. Again, the tradition has been that men satisfy the conditions of such generalizations in that they have long been considered rights owners and rational. Feminists, such as Annette Baier (1992) and Susan Sherwin (1992), call for a reconfiguration of traditional accounts in ethics that tend to elevate men and subordinate women in the ethical life.

Despite notable differences among feminist bioethicists, there are commonalities in their endeavors. These include criticism of the dominant structures, a desire to build more adequate frameworks, and critiques of hierarchical rankings that parcel people into groups based on categories of sex, gender, race, ethnicity, age, disability, genetic predisposition, and other dimensions of difference (Donchin 2009). Tong (1997) argues that the treatments of feminist bioethics offered by feminist bioethicists Susan Sherwin in *No Longer Patient* (1992), Mary Mahowald in *Women and Children in Health Care* (1993), and Susan Wolf and authors in *Feminism and Bioethics* (1996) go some distance toward explaining the need for an "eclectic," "autokoenomous," "positional," and "relational" approach in bioethics. Consider each of these characteristics and how they challenge assumptions in a traditional "gender-neutral" approach in bioethics.

By "eclectic," Tong means "a political framework that permits the use of two or more feminist politics simultaneously, each of them serving as a corrective for the other's myopic tendencies" (Tong 1997, 93). Bringing a number of perspectives to bear on a clinical case that raises ethical concern permits an expansion of the understanding and appreciation of the different views of stakeholders. Women's sexual roles and reproductive responsibilities stressed by care ethicists often combine with women's economic status stressed by power ethicists in ways that put women in a decided disadvantage compared to men. From the perspective of care ethics, one could argue that hormones help women with PMS, menopausal, or post-menopausal symptoms find relief for their debilitating conditions and thus should be made available. From the perspective of power ethics, one could argue that hormones are an arm of a patriarchical culture that seeks to control women, their bodies, and their emotions for the benefit of men and the wallets of male CEOs who run pharmaceutical companies. As a consequence, the wide-spread prescription of hormones to women patients should be critiqued by women for the ways in which they harm women. Acknowledging diverse views provides an opportunity to correct each other's myopic tendencies. There may be good reason to make hormones available to those who seek it and whose conditions are debilitating, but it is incumbent upon the medical community to continue to research the benefits and harms of hormone therapy for women so that women can best be informed about the short-term and long-term effects of the drugs from womb to tomb.

Second, an eclectic view in ethics leads us to reconsider how traditional ethical appeals such as autonomy are understood. For Tong, "autokoenomous," a term drawn from the work of Sarah Lucia Hoagland (1989, 12), means the ability "to use two or more feminist ontologies to better explain the paradox that consists in being a self whose individuality is necessarily constituted through relationships with others" (Tong 1997, 94). The term "autokoenomous" derives from the Greek terms *auto*, meaning "self," and *koinonia*, meaning "community." This contrasts with the principle-based term "autonomy" that derives from the Greek *auto*, meaning "self," and *nomos*, meaning "rule," and refers to an independent, free choice-maker, one who rules himself. The autokoenomous woman "realizes that she is a self inextricably related to other selves" (Tong 1997, 94). This relational account of autonomy receives much attention in the feminist literature and stresses the web of interconnected and sometimes conflicting relationships that inform individuality (see Mackenzie and Stoljar 2000; Friedman 2003). Humans are both individual choice-makers *and* social beings whose selfhood is constituted and maintained within overlapping relationships and communities.

Third, an eclectic view of ethical appeals calls us to be positional in our perspectives. Drawing from Katherine T. Bartlett (1990), Tong defines "positional" as the ability to draw "the line between mere belief (appearance) and true knowledge (reality)" (Tong 1997, 95). Although there is truth to be known, knowledge of this truth is always partial and situational. "[T]ruth is *partial* in that no one individual or group possesses it in entirety" (Tong 1997, 95). Knowledge comes from facts and experiences, but because facts and experiences are inevitably limited, our truths are never total. We cannot be objective enough because we can never see, hear, taste, touch, smell, intuit, or reason enough. As gendered beings who live within particular settings, we rely on each other in order to achieve a wider or more "objective" perspective. And so, "truth is *situated* in that it emerges from the roles and relationships an individual has" (Tong 1997, 95). Biology, along with communities and societies, shape the meaning of our concepts, ideas, and values. Whether menopause is a disintegrating process, a prelude to death, or an integrating experience during which the last and perhaps best chapters of a woman's life are experienced depends on the position one takes.

Fourth, for Tong, just as eclecticism leads to autokoenomy, and autokoenomy leads to positionality, all three of these frameworks lead to some version of a so-called relational ethics (1997, 96). By "relational," Tong means interconnected on the personal as well as collective levels. "[M]ost feminist bioethicists appear to be steering a midcourse between an ethics of care and an ethics of power, each of which is relational in its own way" (Tong 1997, 96). Whereas an ethics of care focuses on microcosmic relationships (e.g., relationships between a particular man and a particular woman), an ethics of power tends to focus on macrocosmic relationships (e.g., relationships between the two genders). "When an ethics of power and an ethics of care combine their moral perspectives, it becomes possible for feminist bioethicists to judge" (Tong 1997, 96) whether the relationship between two individuals is freely chosen or social coerced. Tong gives the example of a relationship between a particular wife and her Alzheimer's-afflicted husband. "On the one hand, if this woman cares for her husband day and night simply because society expects 'good' women to totally subordinate their interests to those of men, her act of 'caring' could border on masochism" (Tong 1997, 96). Alternatively, "if this woman attends to the needs of her ailing spouse because she chooses to do so and in ways that energize rather than enervate her spouse, then her act of caring serves as a self-empowering testament of her love for her husband rather than as evidence of women's subordination to men" (Tong 1997, 96). Here the relational networks that frame an agent's decisions lead to insights into the appropriateness or inappropriateness of the actions.

Tong's emphasis on the need for an eclectic, autokoenomous, positional, and relational approach in bioethics addresses how gender is not simply an import or side-note in bioethical discussions but rather a centralizing theme in bioethics. Gender is centralizing because, as philosopher Susan Bordo puts it, "[o]ne cannot simply be 'human'. . . . Our language, intellectual history, and social forms are 'gendered'; there is no escape from this fact and from its consequences in our lives" (1990, 152). It marks our identity, influences our actions, and serves as the basis for decisions we make in life. In medicine, it represents what we share (being gendered), and how we are different (as gendered beings).

A gender-inclusive approach in bioethics assists us in thinking through some of the ethical implications of gendering disease. An emphasis on the need for an eclectic approach in our bioethical analyses of gender-specific disease will result in varying interpretations of our understanding and use of gender-specific disease, which can be used to forge new perspectives. In assessing the ethicality of how we frame and use gender-specific disease, one will assess how assumptions and claims about women's sexual and gender roles and economic status play out in the clinical description and classification. If there is silence on such claims, or if there is incomplete, inaccurate, or inappropriate assumptions or claims, they can be brought to the surface and reassessed. An eclectic assessment allows for the achievement of a wider perspective on the problem and possible solutions. One might recall the effectiveness and critiques of the women's health movements in forging successful campaigns leading medicine to rethink women's health care in various ways (see Chapter 1). We can say the same about how gender-specific medical voices have been successful in encouraging clinicians to rethink practices in women's health care. Multiple, and at times competing, feminist voices have participated in debates leading to new insights into how to view the problem of gendering disease in alternative ways.

An appreciation of the "autokoenomous" character of autonomy also expands our bioethical analysis of gender-specific disease. Here I think of the work of feminist sociologists of medicine Chloe Bird and Patricia Rieker (2008), who offer an extensive analysis of the need in medicine for a *relational* account of choice that stresses the web of interconnected and sometimes conflicting relationships that affect how medicine views health care disparities. Bird and Rieker develop what they call a "new framework" (2008, 5) for examining gender differences in health based on the sociological view that "constrained choices" affect health, health care, and health policy. They argue that "men's and women's opportunities and choices are to a certain extent constrained by decisions and actions taken by families, employers, communities, and governmental policies. In the long run, these choices can contribute to the observed patterns of gender-based health differences by creating, maintaining, or exacerbating underlying biological differences in health" (Bird and Rieker 2008, 5). Their view is that personal decisions in life are not isolated from the communal and social forces that continually shape them. "Although many of the constraints and their consequences for individual choice are similar for men and women, the health impact will vary somewhat due to differences in both biology and life experiences" (Bird and Rieker 2008, 6). For instance, constrained choices affect men's and women's stress levels differently as they experience competing demands on their time and other resources. This can, in turn, affect their psychological and physical responses to stress, resulting in differences in the expression of disease. This may explain well-documented paradoxes in disease expression, such as why women experience higher rates of depression than men, why men have higher rates of substance abuse and suicide, and why women live on average longer than men. According to Bird and Rieker, researchers and clinicians have only begun to recognize the multiple factors that contribute to disease. "These insights into both men's and women's health produced a new appreciation for the complexity of the paradoxical gender differences in health that challenge more singular notions of the disadvantage or advantage of either gender" (Bird and Rieker 2008, 7).

An emphasis on the "positionality" of our views expands our bioethical analysis of gender-specific disease in that it reminds us of the partial and situated character of knowing and valuing. We learn from this that the quest for gender-neutrality in bioethics and a strictly speaking impartial "objective" human standard involving the elimination of bias is not feasible. According to some feminists (e.g., Harding 1991), some people are in a better position than others to single out problematic ethical occurrences. The thinking, called "standpoint theory," argues that women can have a privileged status. Their experiences as "victims" of discrimination, abuse, and violence lead them to have a vested interest in maintaining the status quo. Those who victimize others produce "distorted visions of the real regularities and underlying causal tendencies in social relations" (Harding 1986, 191). Those who are victims have a stake in changes in the status quo, and their status enables them to see what is wrong with it. In the case of framing gender-specific disease, women patients (and allied health care professionals who are often women) have a privileged status of assessing gender-specific labels and categories because they have long been marginalized in clinical care, in research, and in the profession (Bickel 2000). For this reason women are motivated to criticize "accepted interpretations of reality" (in this case, gender-specific disease labels and categories) and to develop "new and less distorted ways of understanding the world" (Jaggar 1983, 370).

An emphasis on the need for a "relational" approach in our bioethical analysis of gender-specific disease reminds us of lessons from Bird and Rieker (2008) as well as other intersectional thinkers (see Chapter 5). Recall Bird and Rieker's analysis of autonomy as a moral value understood in terms of the agent's interconnected and sometimes conflicting personal and communal relationships as opposed to the individual agent's ability to choose apart from such relations. Attention to the ways that personal, historical, social, cultural, and institutional influences shape medical knowledge reveals "how race, class, gender, and health inequalities are produced within particular social contexts in order to gain a better understanding of commonalities as well as differences in these patterns as they emerge in various locations" (Mullings and Schulz 2006, 7). Applied to a bioethical analysis of framing gender-specific disease, the values under consideration in a bioethical analysis are not separate and distinct from the context of personal and collective relations of the moral agent.

SUMMARY

Assessing ethical considerations raised by our understanding of gender-specific disease involves a reconsideration of the approach we use to analyze them. Following a review of a popular approach used in contemporary bioethics, we find that a gender-neutral principle-based approach in bioethics is insufficient to analyze how medicine frames gender-specific disease. A gender-inclusive intersectional bioethical approach assists in analyzing the unique role gender plays in understanding disease expression and treatment. Reorienting our understanding of gender-specific disease requires that we reorient our bioethical analysis as well.

8 Integrative Bioethics and Assessing Gender-Specific Disease

GENDER-INCLUSIVITIES

The critiques of bioethics forwarded by Tong (1997) and other feminist bioethicists have the advantage of leading us to reevaluate what bioethical methodology we use to assess the ethical implications of understanding gender-specific disease. Indeed this makes sense. Why would anyone assess a gender matter with a gender-neutral perspective? Nevertheless, we need to be cautious here. Relying on the lessons we have learned from integrative thinking in Chapter 5 and 6, and gender-inclusive bioethics in Chapter 7, this chapter further develops the need for an integrative approach in bioethics on matters concerning gender-specific disease. It draws from my previous work with philosopher of science Raphael Sassower (2007) to show that a gender-inclusive bioethical approach will need to be integrative in order to assess how we frame gender-specific disease. If the bioethical approach is not integrative, it will miss the mark on properly framing gender, disease, and their relations. The chapter extends this lesson by providing a case-study analysis of gender-specific AIDS. It concludes with some general suggestions regarding what normative concerns to watch for as medicine moves to develop accounts of gender-specific disease.

TOWARD AN INTEGRATIVE BIOETHICS

As reviewed in the previous chapter, a gender-inclusive approach in bioethics represents an important step in helping to assess the ethical implications of framing gender-specific disease. In matters concerning gender-specific disease, we would expect that our bioethical analyses pay special attention to how gender, disease, and their relation are understood. As we have learned, gender is not a fixed, stable factor that a person "has." It is a dimension of analysis that intersects with other dimensions, such as biological phenomena, experience, assumed roles, self-attributions, race/ethnicity, class, lifestyle, age, etc. Disease and disease causation are integrative as well. Our understanding of disease is far from a simple thing out there to be discovered. It entails symptomatic, etiological, and multi-factorial accounts of clinical phenomena that serve as treatment warrants. Our understanding of disease causation is far from a simple linear relation between cause and effect. It involves a host of ways to understand how disease comes about and how it can be treated. In the end, gender-specific disease is a gender-inclusive integrative notion. It brings together a range of explanations and interventions for clinical problems that patients bring to the attention of health care professionals.

Given that gender-specific disease is integrative, any analysis of its bio-ethical implications will need to be integrative as well. A gender-inclusive non-integrative bioethics approach will miss important issues raised by how we know and employ an integrative concept. If the gender-inclusive bioethical account is not integrative, if it depicts, or is used to depict, gender as a static independent patient identifier or it resists intersecting with other gender-neutral positions, it will not be able to uncover problematic assumptions and claims about gender-specific disease. Indeed, insofar as a gender-inclusive approach is integrative, it serves our purposes well. The gender-inclusive approach to analyzing ethical issues in medicine developed by intersectional feminists comes to mind. We'll explore the need for a gender-inclusive integrative approach in bioethics in what follows.

In *Ethical Choices in Contemporary Medicine*, philosopher of science Raphael Sassower and I (2007) develop an initial account of an integrative bioethical approach in medicine. We elucidate some of the prominent epistemological and ethical frameworks in philosophical and medical discourse in order to bring about a deeper appreciation of the different approaches and responses that frame debates on disease, including the bioethical ones. We analyze various contemporary bioethical debates about health care provision as it relates to socio-cultural assumptions that impact diagnosis and prognosis, from cancer to AIDS, and from mainstream to alternative clinical procedures regarding end-of-life care. We find that each clinical choice made in medicine shifts radically from being justified exclusively as a scientifically based choice to a more nuanced explanation of what might be useful under specific sets of circumstances. In the end, Sassower and I call for an integrative approach in contemporary bioethical discourse: "Integrative bioethics embeds bioethical reflection in a confluence of disciplines that provide an appreciation of different aspects of medical practice and bring into view different concerns and possible pathways for intervening to address health care needs" (Sassower and Cutter 2007, 1). It is a reflection not only of the need to "mainstream" so-called "alternative" accounts in bioethics (a category in which "feminist bioethics" typically appears), but of the philosophical insight that *a* definitive approach in bioethics (including a feminist one) is unavailable.

Current practice in bioethics is marked by numerous, and, at times, competing approaches. The principle-based and gender-inclusive-based ones reviewed in the previous chapter are just a small selection of the options. Although I will not cover all the approaches here, readers can pick up encyclopedic entries to obtain a sense of the range of views in bioethics currently being supported (see, for example, entries in *Encyclopedia of Bioethics*, *Stanford Encyclopedia of Philosophy*). A brief sense of the range of views follows in order to support my view that a gender-inclusive integrative bioethical approach to matters concerning gender-specific disease makes much needed sense.

The terrain of positions in contemporary bioethics is expansive. In addition to a principle-based approach in bioethics (see Chapter 6), there are numerous critiques of principle-based positions (Sassower and Cutter 2007, 128ff). Dominant ones to come on the scene in the last twenty-five years are casuistry, virtue ethics, contemporary sentient theory, global ethics, communitarianism, pragmatism, and narrative (or discourse) bioethics. Casuistrists (e.g., Jonsen and Toulmin 1988) hold that induction (reasoning from particular cases to general norms about cases) is superior to deduction (reasoning from general norms to particular cases). Induction allows the facts of a case to speak for themselves, so to speak, allowing us to see if these particular facts justify exceptions to the general norms which deductivists tend to use. Virtue ethicists (e.g., MacIntyre 1981) see right action as flowing out of one's character. Upbringing, education, the example of others, reflection, personal effort, and experience all play important roles in the ability to pursue the right and the good. Sentient theorists (e.g., Singer 1995) focus on sentiments or emotions and hold that people who feel altruistic emotions have the ability to perform altruistic actions. This view underlies Jeremy Bentham's famous statement: "The question is not, Can they *reason*? Nor, Can they *talk*? But, Can they *suffer*?" (1996, 311). Global bioethicists (e.g., United Nations 2004) focus on the non-exclusionary values that humans share across border and nations, and seek to enhance the expression of such values in human practices. In these discussions, the achievement of physical and mental health is a central moral goal. Communitarians view bioethics as a group project (e.g., ten Have and Keasberry 1992) and emphasize the responsibility of the community to the individual, and the individual's responsibility to the community, where "community" may or may not mean "society" in general. Pragmatists (e.g., Moreno 1995, 2003) place importance on the context of deliberation, and the conversation, which is crucial for all modes of representing experience. Because this context is typically social, a pragmatist emphasizes the interpersonal dimension as crucial for all modes of representing experience. Narrative (communicative or discourse) bioethicists (e.g., Brody 1994) emphasize the narration of the stories of people's particular lives and what we can learn from these.

In addition, we are reminded from the last chapter that feminist bioethical contributions have made their distinctive mark in contemporary bioethical discussions in their different ways (Tong 1997, 87–88). Some have more naturalized (or rational-empirical) epistemological commitments, some more social constructivist ones, and some more postmodern ones. Naturalized feminist bioethicists (Antony 2002) subscribe to objective, impartial, neutral, and universal standards of behavior and often look to the sciences in order to establish an empirical basis for their claims. Social constructionists (e.g., Harding 1991) hold that medicine is not so objective and impartial, but is rather androcentric. In order to assess the "facts" of medicine, physicians need to listen to women's narratives and take seriously the somatic and psychological complaints that individual women bring into the clinic. Privileging the clinician as authority in medical knowledge fails to take into consideration that medical knowledge involves more than "bench scientific" facts about diseases. Postmodernists (e.g., Alcoff 2006) tend to hold that epistemology is really ideology and that there is no such thing as objective knowledge, regardless of the standpoint. Any attempt to develop "objective" knowledge mimics the kind of universalistic, absolutivist, deductivist thought that suggests that there is only one way to tell a story about reality.

Divergent views in bioethics remind us about how our conversations usually go, and how they are filled with various and differing views of the world, knowledge, and values. In the case of entertaining different bioethical approaches to assessing how we gender disease, we can say that some have been better at focusing on the role gender plays in medical knowledge and practice (e.g., gender-inclusive bioethics), whereas others do worse because of their silence on the issue (e.g., principle-based approach). Others are successful in resolving conflicts in an efficient manner (e.g., the principle-based approaches in which ethical principles are applied to particular cases), whereas others have had the advantage of focusing on the particulars in a case (e.g., bioethical casuistry). Some have provided robust unification (e.g., the principle-based approach), whereas others are skeptical about such possibility (e.g., postmodern feminist bioethics). Some make the claim that certain features of their position are non-negotiable (e.g., a libertarian principle-based bioethics), whereas others recognize the negotiability of their assertions (e.g., discourse bioethics). Some work better with religious or spiritual matters in medicine (e.g., a religious bioethics), whereas others have little to say about such topics (e.g., secular bioethics).

An integrative bioethics offers a way to talk about approaches in bioethics that are epistemologically and axiologically heterogenous and useful for our purposes. The lesson is to see such approaches as evolving and relational bodies of knowledge and values set within particular historical and cultural contexts. In this way, the relations, intersections, and interplays discussed in the prior chapters involving discovery and creation, description and evaluation, knowing and valuing, facts and values, and diagnosis and treatment are theoretically and practically fruitful in so far as they reflect how we know and intervene in medicine. Although there are good reasons to hold as insufficient a gender-neutral analysis of gender-inclusive matters, one can expect to find a range of analyses. The accounts we give in medicine will in the end be multi-faceted, diverse, and dynamic, as they take into consideration the complexity of human conditions, the character of gender-specific disease, and the ways we evaluate ethical indiscretions.

The integrative bioethical approach that is supported here shares similarities with the heterogeneity of the "expressive collaborative" method developed by feminist moral philosopher Margaret Urban Walker (1998, 2003). Walker's expressive collaborative method "prescribes an investigation of morality as a socially embodied medium of mutual understanding and negotiation between people over their responsibility for things open to human care and response" (1998, 9). In other words, for Walker, morality is expressed in interpersonal contexts; it "arises out of and is reproduced or modified in what goes on between or among people" (1998, 10). Moreover, it is collaborative in the sense that "we construct and sustain it together" (1998, 10), although not always in chosen or equal terms.

The expressive collaborative method of moral inquiry consists of four characteristics. First, "morality occurs in real human practices, and we need to try and understand these practices in the social contexts in which they occur" (1998, 16). To understand moral phenomena, then, it will be important to engage in descriptive analysis of how moral agency occurs and how it is formed in interpersonal and shared social contexts. Secondly, "the practices characteristic of morality are practices of responsibility" (1998, 16), where responsibility is a prescriptive notion probing what ought to be done in certain situations. Thirdly, "morality is not socially modular" (1998, 17); in other words, morality is not composed of standardized social units or sections for easy construction or flexible arrangement. Moral concepts and practices are intersectional and framed in terms of dimensions of analysis. Lastly, and as a consequence of the first three assumptions, "[m]oral theorizing and moral epistemology need to be freed from the impoverishing legacies of ideality and purity that make most people's moral lives disappear, or render those lives unintelligible" (1998, 18). Morality is embedded in actual human practices that do not operate alone.

Walker's expressive collaborative model is thus a philosophical model that gives an interpretation of the moral life that functions both descriptively and prescriptively. Descriptively, the aim is to give an interpretation and/or reveal what is "morality." This description can entail "an empirically saturated reflective analysis of what is going on in actual moral orders" (Walker 1998, 11) and it can entail "many different kinds of factual researches, including documentary, historical, psychological, ethnographic, and sociological ones" (Walker 1998, 11). Prescriptively, the aim is to provide guidelines for some of the important purposes of morality and the practices on which it depends, for better or worse.

The integrative approach suggested in this project finds similarities with the expressive collaborative method. In Chapter 2, we considered the descriptive role of gender-specific medical claims as expressed in real clinical practices. In Chapter 3, we explored the prescriptive or normative implications of describing gender-specific disease. Chapter 4 bridged the descriptive and prescriptive role of gender-specific disease and showed their interrelations within particular contexts. Chapters 5 and 6 echoed that the descriptive and prescriptive roles of gender-specific disease are not socially modular. Chapter 7 introduced the need for an integrative bioethical approach to gender-specific disease. Gender-specific disease and related bioethical analyses are integrative, or as Walker would say, expressive and collaborative. It interprets as well as evaluates our descriptive and prescriptive commitments within particular contexts. In short, Walker's suggestions are given support in this analysis for the ways in which we might free moral theorizing, in this case on matters concerning how we understand gender-specific disease, from the legacies of ideality and purity, and embed analyses of our understanding and use of gender-specific disease within everyday practices in medicine and in bioethical analyses.

CASE STUDY OF GENDER-SPECIFIC AIDS

We now take a look at how an integrative bioethical approach is needed to uncover problematic assumptions and claims about gender-specific disease. Consider an integrative bioethical analysis of framing AIDS as a gender-specific disease (an extension of what is found in Sassower and Cutter 2007, 13ff). If one is assessing AIDS as a gender-specific disease, one will have to consider the contexts in which discussions occur. Is one talking about a particular disease as conceived in the early 1980s, the late 1980s, or the early 2000s? Recall that in the early 1980s, and after subsequent discussions, AIDS referred to a set of signs and symptoms such as high fever, skin blotches, and unintentional weight loss (Centers for Disease Control 1981a, 1981b, 1982). It was considered a "gay disease." It was not until the late 1980s that AIDS came to be understood through an etiological framework involving the viral entity called HIV, the name of which was arrived at by a consensus group after lengthy discussion about what was known about this viral entity and what language would best fit clinical discourse (Varmus 1989). Research in the 1990s established that HIV is not a simple entity but one that mutates. It did not act alone but rather acted in concert with certain features of the cell to penetrate and replicate at levels that lead to the signs and symptoms associated with HIV infection. Certain behaviors (e.g., anal, but not oral, sex) were seen to be conducive to an increase in HIV infection (National Institute of Allergy and Infectious Diseases 1995). In the 1990s, and in contexts in which women were treated largely as sexual objects, HIV infections among women rose quickly. Therefore, AIDS comes to be understood as a multi-factorial phenomenon, one in which internal etiological and external environmental factors dually operate. Recognition of gender-specific differences in how HIV was contracted and expressed fueled research on women with AIDS (Goldsmith 1992). Increasingly it became evident that women were particularly vulnerable to heterosexual transmission of HIV due to substantial mucosal exposure to seminal fluids. This biological fact amplified the risk of HIV transmission when coupled with a high prevalence of non-consensual sex, sex without condom use, and the unknown and/or high-risk behaviors of HIV-infected partners. Manifestations of HIV disease particular to women, such as recurrent yeast infections, severe pelvic inflammatory change in the cervix, and increased rates of cervical cancer became notable. As we can see, much depends on the context of the descriptive claims made about AIDS as a gender-specific disease.

Note how the treatment offered to a patient turns on how a gender-specific disease is defined by researchers and clinicians. In the early years of the AIDS epidemic, cold compresses and topical ointments were recommended to all regardless of gender to calm the fever and soothe skin irritations. In the late 1980s and early 1990s, clinical researchers began the hunt for anti-retroviral therapy, pharmaceutical agents that prevent HIV from infecting cells or stop it from replicating in the body (Gallo and Montagnier 1987; Fauci 1993; Klatt 1998). Early recommendations focused mainly on gay practices. In the early to late 1990s, public health recommendations regarding safe sex practices and AIDS prevention became commonplace. Attention began to be paid to the plight of women as sexual objects and victims of incest and rape (Faden 1996). More attention was given to making available condoms and information on the toll which unprotected sex was taking on women. Research began to emerge that women responded differently to antiretroviral therapies, and that women needed to be treated earlier than men in the course of the disease. Others saw poverty, and not HIV, as responsible for AIDS (Duesberg 1994), and recommended increased dollars for public health initiatives and an increased provision of basic needs (e.g., food, shelter, and health care). Still others were on the hunt for an immunization against HIV infection (Fauci 1993). Treatment recommendations turn out to be linked to how gender-specific disease is defined.

Not only is our understanding of a gender-specific disease related to its treatment, but bioethical discourse about rights, welfare, justice, oppression, care, and power will inevitably reflect how we describe and treat a gender-specific problem. If one understands AIDS as a constellation of signs and symptoms (Centers for Disease Control 1982), then much attention will be paid to changing the signs and symptoms and reducing patient symptoms in order to promote patient welfare and care for the patient. Alternatively, if one understands AIDS in terms of an etiological entity (Gallo and Montagnier 1987), a fair amount of focus will be on what and who is responsible for the spread of HIV infection and what can be done to prevent against this. The bioethical focus becomes the duty humans have to prevent harm and the rights held by victims to be protected against unconsensual harm. Then again, if one understands AIDS in terms of gender-specific factors, much attention will be paid to the gender factors that bring the gender-specific conditions about. The bioethical focus becomes gender-inclusive, focusing on how patient welfare, choice, and access to medical knowledge and care are constituted, promoted, and/or compromised as a result of gender status. It is tied to how medicine frames its diagnostics and treatments as a reflection of its understanding of gender, sex, disease, and disease condition. The recognition of the multi-dimensional character of knowing and treating in medicine is met with a multi-dimensional way of addressing the bioethical issues that are raised.

On this interpretation, resolution of a bioethical conflict depends on the methodology one brings to the conflict resolution along with the clinical descriptions and prescriptions one adopts. This is certainly the case in the context of knowing and treating AIDS. If one is committed to a principle-based account of autonomy, as are Beauchamp and Childress (2009), one will seek to ensure an individual's right to hold views, to make choices, to have his of her welfare promoted, and to be a recipient of just actions. If one embraces a gender-inclusive account of autonomy, as Tong (1997, 94) and others (Bird and Rieker 2008) call us to do, one will be in the business of mapping out the gendered choices operating in the case to appreciate their intersectional character in light of other dimensions of analysis. One is reminded of the challenges in the early years of the epidemic to encourage medicine to attend to the plight and growing numbers of HIV-infected women. It was no longer sufficient simply to recognize a woman's right to information about AIDS and expect changes in the number of HIV-infected women. It was no longer sufficient simply to recognize that unprotected sex can be harmful to women. Actions that promoted change in women's sexual, cultural, and institutional lives were seen to be medically necessary on grounds that there exists oppressive cultural and institutional forces that fuel how women's choices are made and constrained, and how women's health is compromised. The bioethical analysis we give reflects how we understand the problem, and how we understand the problem leads us to embrace particular bioethical approaches over others.

An integrative bioethical case study of framing AIDS as a gender-specific condition can offer a wide range of perspectives on the bioethical challenges that arise when framing gender-specific disease. Whether it is gender-specific AIDS or heart disease, we will want to attend to the context of the gender-specific disease, the relation between understanding and treating the gender-specific disease, and the methodological assumptions and claims framing our ethical judgments of the gender-specific disease. Special attention will be needed on how gender (and sex), disease, and their relation are understood in such contexts.

NORMATIVE CONSIDERATIONS

Guided by integrative thinking, consider some of the ethical considerations to watch for as gender-specific nosologies and nosographies are developed.

There are certainly a number of considerations that could be addressed, but I'll focus mainly on three general ways of assessing ethical implications of the ways in which gender-specific disease is understood in light of what we have learned in the previous chapters. These include the need (a) to uncover the use of gender-specific descriptions and prescriptions that harm members of particular genders in medicine, (b) to assess gender-specific harms in health care practice and research that reflect problems in gender-specific descriptions and prescriptions, and (c) to critique additional sources of harms that lead to problems in gender-specific descriptions and prescriptions and/or harms in practice or research. The list reflects some of the topics raised in this study and serves as examples of ethical concerns to watch for as medicine moves to gender disease.

A preliminary note is in order about harm. It is the harm of the clinical condition that is the primary focus of medicine's efforts to understand and change a clinical condition. Here harm has to do with being "unable to exercise the capacities that constitute our good" (Kaufman 1997, 281). Through pharmaceutical, surgical, and palliative interventions, medicine offers the opportunity for patients to exercise such capacities, such as freedom of action and physical achievement, the normal range of which can be empirically established. Determining what constitutes harm in medicine is a complex endeavor. Philosophically speaking, much depends on whose harm is at stake, and how and why. Is the concern an individual patient or a community? Is the focus the harm of a woman, man, child, or fetus? Is the concern the harm of members of a certain racial or economic group? Is it on public health considerations and the need to contain an epidemic? Is it on budgetary considerations and the need to contain costs? Is it on health policy or legal considerations and the need to maintain consistency in these areas? Is it on a host of these factors and their interrelations? Disagreement within seemingly similar standpoints or perspectives is easy to find so that once again the choice or selection of the context of the harms under consideration is itself at stake. This is not a plea for understanding and classifying harms by referendum or town meeting. This is instead the claim that choices among different understandings of harm within medicine are matters of collaboration that have implications in bioethical analysis.

Consider three types of normative considerations raised by gendering disease. First, integrative bioethical approaches to gender-specific disease encourage that we question the use of gender-specific descriptions and prescriptions that perpetuate harms against members of particular genders. This is to encourage critically analyzing gender-specific descriptions and prescriptions in order to uncover problematic assumptions, evidence, and methodologies that result in practices that harm women. In the previous chapters, we have seen particular examples of gender-specific clinical categories that lead to practices in medicine that harm women. These include those that fail to take into account gender as a variable in disease expression and treatment, as found in our case study of AIDS. These also include those that have inappropriate conceptions of gender as causally linked to disease, as found in our case study of menopause as a disease.

Further, we are encouraged to look for cases of undergeneralization, overgeneralization, and mislabeling of clinical conditions that affect members of particular genders. There is much work that can be done here. Which clinical conditions currently recognized in medicine have minimal to no discussion of the gender-specific factors that may operate? The lack of gender-specific pediatric issues on the American Academy of Pediatrics website comes to mind. What clinical conditions currently recognized in medicine are assumed to be gender-specific, that is, are assumed to be expressed primarily by women, men, lesbians, gays, transgenders, and bisexuals when there is evidence that the assumptions are incorrect? Although depression is certainly evidence among women, men also experience it. What gender-specific clinical conditions currently recognized in medicine can we say are mislabeled?

A general suggestion put forth in this inquiry regarding assessing gender-specific descriptions and prescriptions is to unroot problematic assumptions in descriptions and prescriptions by asking whether there would be differences in clinical diagnosis, clinical treatment, clinical research, clinical curriculum, clinical policy, and health care delivery if the patients or research subjects were women (Nobelius and Wainer 2004, 14–15). As we have learned, medicine has embraced since the beginning, and despite Hippocrates' (2005 [fifth c. B.C.E.], 62) advice, a gender-neutral perspective of patients. To incorporate a gender-inclusive perspective is to acknowledge the differential roles that gender plays in disease expression and treatment and the ways in which the gender of the health care practitioner influences a health care event and clinical texts and teaching styles. How would the diagnoses, prognoses, treatments, medical evidence, anatomical sketches, guidelines, laws, and/or health care access be different if the players were women? One's answers to these queries may signal areas in need of further investigation and revision in gender-specific medicine, especially if the investigation reveals that there are harms that occur as a result of not taking gender properly into consideration.

Second, an integrative approach encourages that we assess gender-specific harms in health care research and therapy that reflect problems in such descriptions and prescriptions. Often clinicians, researchers, patients, and concerned parties take for granted the descriptions and prescriptions that are employed in medicine because they think they are non-negotiable and do not fully appreciate the assumptions and claims that go into making clinical categories. In assessing gender-specific descriptions and prescriptions, it may be easier to note health care harms and then move to question the descriptions and prescriptions that contribute to justifying such harms. For instance, an increase in numbers of HIV infection among women led to rethinking how AIDS was understood. An increase in breast and endometrial cancers led to questioning standard remedies for menopausal symptom.

In the face of health care harms, we reflect on the assumptions and claims that frame how gender-specific disease is understood and treated and how they contribute to fostering such harms.

We have already seen how a focus on harm leads to a reconsideration of the clinical descriptions and prescriptions that operate. One could say that this was a major impetus behind the women's health movements of the latter twenty-first century. When patient reports and clinical investigations showed that harms occurred because of a lack of accurate diagnoses and treatments, attention was often given to particular medical practices, including the assumptions and language used in the practices. The harms brought about by widely prescribed hormone therapies for women, inaccurate diagnoses of heart attacks among women, and the overuse of cesarean sections among women all have contributed to a rethinking of descriptions and prescriptions in medicine.

Third, an integrative bioethical approach to gender-specific disease encourages that we critique additional sources of harm that lead to problems in clinical descriptions and prescriptions and/or harms toward members of particular genders in health care. Here one might start with sources of harm that affect members of a particular gender and reflect on how they contribute to errant disease descriptions and prescriptions and/or health care practices. Of particular interest today is the role of poverty in disease and health status. According to a 2006 report (United Nations Development 2006), Norway has the highest level of human development and Niger the lowest. Here level of human development is a composite of three dimensions of development that correlate with poverty and in turn, disease and illness: living a long and healthy life (measured by life expectancy), being educated (measured by adult literacy and enrollment in primary, secondary, and tertiary schools), and having a decent standard of living (measured by purchasing power and income). Individuals in Norway are nearly fifty times wealthier and live almost twice as long as those in Niger and have nearly universal enrollment in education, compared with 21% in Niger. People in the thirty-one countries with the lowest levels of human development, which represent 9% of the population, have an average life expectancy of forty-six years, thirty-two years less than in countries with the highest levels of human development. This discrepancy illustrates something that most of us are already familiar with: that poverty prevents individuals from attaining education and employment, escaping poverty, achieving and maintaining health, and managing disease, illness, and disability (also see Flanagin and Winkler 2006; World Health Organization 2007; Blumenthal and Kagan 2002).

Tied to the problem of poverty and of particular significance in women's health care is the role of violence in bringing about and sustaining disease and illness among women. According to the Centers for Disease Control and Prevention, "[v]iolence is a serious public health problem in the U.S. From infants to the elderly, it affects people in all stages of life. In 2007, more than 18,000 people were victims of homicide and more than 34,000 took their own life" (Centers for Disease Control 2011, 1). In addition to the number of violent deaths, "[m]any more survive violence and are left with permanent physical and emotional scars. Violence also erodes communities by reducing productivity, decreasing property values, and disrupting social services" (Centers for Disease Control 2011, 1). Women are particularly vulnerable to the negative effects of violence because they are typically less able physically to defend themselves against it, less able to move away from it because of socio-economic constraints, and less able to change it because of lack of educational opportunities in certain cultures. Violence under-mines somatic and psychological welfare and contributes to an increase in lack of social participation, employment, and education.

Physician Claudia Garcia-Moreno and colleagues studied the extent of physical and sexual partner violence against 24,097 women in fifteen sites in ten countries: Bangladesh, Brazil, Ethiopia, Japan, Namibia, Peru, Samoa, Serbia and Montenegro, Thailand, and the United Republic of Tan-zania. They found that "[t]he reported lifetime prevalence of physical or sexual partner violence, or both, varied from 15% to 71%, with two sites having a prevalence of less than 25%, seven between 25% and 50%, and six between 50% and 75%. Between 4% and 54% of respondents reported physical or sexual partner violence, or both, in the past year" (Garcia-Moreno et al. 2006, 1). They further found that "[m]en who were more controlling were more likely to be violent against their partners. In all but one setting women were at far greater risk of physical or sexual violence by a partner than from violence by other people" (Garcia-Moreno et al. 2006, 1). Their findings confirm "that physical and sexual partner vio-lence against women is widespread. The variation in prevalence within and between settings highlights that this violence in not inevitable, and must be addressed" (Garcia-Moreno et al. 2006, 1).

Their work with patients leads health care practitioners to appreciate that large-scale social forces, such as poverty and violence, often deter-mine who falls ill and who has access to care. For practitioners of public health, the social determinants of disease are even harder to disregard. But, as physician and anthropologist Paul Farmer and his co-authors put it, "[u]nfortunately, this awareness is seldom translated into formal frameworks that link social analysis to everyday clinical practice. One reason for this gap is that the holy grail of modern medicine remains the search for the molecular basis of disease" (Farmer et al. 2006). Although studies on the molecular basis of disease have certainly benefited patients, "exclusive focus on molecular-level phenomena has contributed to the increasing 'desocialization' of scientific inquiry: a tendency to ask only biological questions about what are in fact *biosocial* phenomena" (Farmer et al. 2006). According to Farmer and his colleagues, a greater biosocial understanding of medical phenomena is needed. "Social analysis, how-ever rudimentary, occurs at the bedside, in the clinic, in field sites, and in the margins of the biomedical literature" (Farmer et al. 2006). It is to be found, for example, in any significant survey of adherence to therapy for chronic diseases, in studies of what were once termed "social diseases" such as venereal disease and tuberculosis (TB), and in the phenomenon of acquired resistance to antibiotics. Such examples lead Farmer and his colleagues to ask: "Can we speak of the 'natural history' of any of these diseases without addressing social forces, including racism, pollution, poor housing, and poverty, that shape their course in both individuals and populations? Does our clinical practice acknowledge what we already know—namely, that social and environmental forces will limit the effectiveness of our treatments?" (Farmer et al. 2006).

SUMMARY

An integrative bioethical approach to gender-specific disease encourages that we view ethical issues through integrated contexts. It recognizes the strengths and relevance of a gender-inclusive bioethical approach in assessing gender-specific disease. It integrates those strengths into an approach that acknowledges the need for an integrative bioethical approach to gender-specific disease. An integrative approach attends to the connections among how we know and treat disease, health disparities, and the contexts in which these are framed in gender-specific medicine. In the end, it offers a both/and emphasis on context and integration in relation to a bioethical analysis of gender-specific disease.

9 Implications for Health Care for Men, Children, and Members of the LGBT Communities

GENDER-SPECIFIC MEDICINE IS NOT JUST ABOUT WOMEN

This study focuses largely on women's health care as a major case study of the character of gender-specific disease. Nevertheless, reflections on the character of gender-specific disease carry implications for health care involving those other than women. What follows shares some of these implications for health care for men, children, and members of the lesbian, gay, bisexual, and transgender communities. It draws from the reflections of Demetrius Porche (2007), Kandyce Larson et al. (2008), and the Institute of Medicine (2001a) on the need for gender-specific research and practice in areas that focus on those other than women.

IMPLICATIONS FOR MEN'S HEALTH CARE

At first blush, there appears to be plenty of attention given to men's health and therefore little need for an analogous "men's health movement" in health care. One could say that the history of medicine has been a men's health movement. Up until the 1980s, physicians in the U.S. have traditionally been male. Anatomical sketches in clinical textbooks have traditionally been based on the male body. Men have been involved in clinical research since its inception and there have been all kinds of reasons tied to reproductive concerns to exclude females. There has been no shortage of studies involving men on cardiac disease. Men have traditionally been involved in the development and administration of medicine and science since the beginning and therefore have had greater say in these areas and on what should be funded and studied (see Chapter 1).

On second thought, there are reasons to claim that more attention is needed on men's health and better ways to deliver health care to men. According to the National Center for Health Care Statistics (2008b, 2008c), men experience more cancers and accidents than women. They experience different signs and symptoms in depression and heart disease. According to the Department of Health and Human Services (2006), 20% of men surveyed reported not regularly seeking clinical services and 26% reported not having seen a physician or health care professional in the previous twelve months. Although hospital stays for men are generally fewer than for women, men report experiencing an average of three bed days because of illness or injury, which translates into lost workdays. Perhaps of greatest concern is that men have a 41% chance of dying earlier than women and their life expectancy is about 5.3 years less than women (Centers for Disease Control and Prevention 2006).

There are reasons, then, to look at the implications of an integrative approach to gender-specific disease on men's health care. A study of how men's diseases are understood reveals some claims and assumptions about men that may be challenged. In the previous chapters, we considered how medicine's silence on how AIDS affected women led to a lack of proper care of women in medicine. An analogous example in men's health care might be depression. With regard to depression, more than six million men in the U.S. have been diagnosed with depression (National Institutes of Mental Health 2008). Diamond (2004) argues that there are many more men who experience depression who are not diagnosed. New research shows that work stress and job strain are linked to significant depression and anxiety in men (Cleveland Clinic 2008). Some of the reasons that the symptoms of depression in men go unnoticed include that men tend to deny having coping problems because they are supposed to be "strong" or "tough." Further, the symptoms of depression in men differ from the symptoms found in women (Cleveland Clinic 2008). Where women typically cry or verbally express interest in suicide when depressed (but usually do not carry this out), men typically keep their feelings hidden and become more irritable, seek reliance on alcohol or substances, and/or become aggressive. The stereotype that "men do not get down" or that "men are not emotional" leads men not to seek advice from health care professionals and health care professionals not to diagnose men with depression (Cleveland Clinic 2008). One result is much higher suicide rates in the U.S. for males compared to females, where suicide is the seventh leading cause of death in males (resulting in 26,308 deaths) and the sixteenth leading cause of death in females (resulting in 6,992 deaths) (Heron 2010, 9).

Whereas men may be underdiagnosed with depression, there is evidence that they are overdiagnosed with erectile dysfunction. Erectile dysfunction is a clinical category that emerged in the 1990s and has received a great deal of attention in the U.S. market, especially through advertisements by drug companies offering promises to correct the disorder. The Mayo Clinic (2008) reports one in ten men experience an inability to develop and maintain erection of the penis. The National Kidney and Urologic Disease Information Clearinghouse (2008) reports that erectile dysfunction affects fifteen to thirty million American men, which translates into one-fifth of all American men. Pfizer, the developer of Viagra, the most popular medication for erectile dysfunction, reports that "more than half of all men over 40 have some difficulty getting and maintaining an erection" (Pfizer 2008, 1). Such differences in the number of those affected indicate some disagreement or confusion over the clinical criteria for such a condition. (Or, cynically speaking, it indicates the interest on the part of Pfizer to sell Viagra.) Viagra was patented in 1996 and approved by the FDA in 1998. Sales for the product totaled over $1 billion dollars between 1999 and 2001. In 2004, global sales for Viagra, and its rivals Cialis and Levitra, were $2.5 billion (Berenson 2005). It is interesting to note that only 25% of Viagra is prescribed by Board Certified urologists (National Kidney and Urologic Disease Information Clearinghouse 2008). Current emphasis on erectile dysfunction tells us something about the priorities in men's health care.

Certainly more can be said about how men and their diseases are understood in medicine on par with the more extensive analysis found in the earlier chapters on women's health care. But this is a matter for another time. Suffice it to say that men need a men's health movement. Compared with the women's health movement, the men's health movement in the U.S. has been a limited endeavor. The so-called "men's health movement" began to organize in the U.S. in the 1990s. According to Demetrius Porche (2007), this movement is in part a response to the growing women's health movement and in part a response to lack of attention to what defines men's health. In the U.S., the Men's Health Network was founded in 1992 and the *American Journal of Men's Health,* which is published though the Louisiana State University of Health Science Center School of Nursing, was founded in March of 2007 (Porche 2007). The European-based *Journal of Men's Health and Gender* (now called *Journal of Men's Health*) began publishing through Elsevier in 2004. Then there is the popular magazine *Men's Health Magazine*, published by Rodale, Inc., which focuses primarily on body building and male sexual responses, thus fulfilling some of the stereotypes about men raised above.

Gender-specific medicine would be wise to heed Porche's call for a broader sense of men's health in order to redefine the dialogue and move men's health in productive directions (Porche and Willis 2004). Gender-specific medicine has an opportunity to develop new models of diagnosis, prognosis, and treatment for conditions that uniquely affect men. It has the opportunity to challenge assumptions and claims about men and the diseases that particularly affect them as it adopts new nomenclature and taxonomies in men's health care. As we learned in Chapter 6, the categories of "male" and "man" already assume a structure of clinical reality and we may not be able to rethink the assumptions and claims that frame the categories without changing the categories or lenses themselves. Men's health care might consider moving beyond the language of "male" and "men" and use the language of underlying genotypical and phenotypical factors that contribute to the conditions that patients bring to the attention of health care professionals. Rethinking the assumptions and claims made about being "male" or "man" in medicine will influence how medicine thinks about men's diseases and how gender contributes to disease expression and treatment. In the end, reflection upon the character of gender-specific disease has implications in men's health care.

IMPLICATIONS FOR PEDIATRIC HEALTH CARE

Another group that goes underrepresented in this study is children. At first blush there appears to be plenty of attention given to girls and boys. When the American Academy of Pediatrics (AAP) was established in 1930, the idea that children have special developmental and health needs was a new one. Preventive health practices now associated with child care, such as immunizations and regular health exams, were only just beginning to change the custom of treating children as "miniature adults." Today the AAP has over 60,000 physicians as members and continues to work toward educating health care professionals about the special needs of children (American Academy of Pediatrics 2011). It oversees the academic journal *Pediatrics*, which started in 1948, and continues to rally for improvements in assessing quality improvement in child health services (Beal et al. 2004), especially in the areas of immunizations and regular health exams.

In addition, today the federal-state financing systems for Medicaid and the State Children's Health Insurance Program provide a significant amount of money to pediatric care. Medicaid is the largest children's health program in the U.S. and covers 29.5 million children. In 1997, under President Clinton, the Children's Health Insurance Program (CHIP) was established to provide coverage for children who did not qualify for Medicaid, but whose families could not afford private insurance. This legislation, which has cost over $10 billion dollars since 1997, has reduced the rate of uninsured low-income children by almost one third, from 23% to 7.6% (Stein and Silverstein 2010).

Still, there are numerous needs in pediatric health care. There could always be more funds. Bethell et al. report that "[a]n estimated 43% of US children (32 million) currently have at least 1 of 20 chronic health conditions assessed, increasing to 54.1% when overweight, obesity, or being at risk for developmental delays are included" (2011, S22). Compared with privately insured children, "the prevalence, complexity, and severity of health problems were systematically greater for the 29.1% of all children who are publicly insured children after adjusting for variations in demographic and socioeconomic factors" (Bethell et al. 2011, S22). More attention is needed on how to deliver better health care to children, especially those who struggle with ADHD, asthma, autism, obesity, violence that impacts health, and access to health care (American Academy of Pediatrics 2011). In addition, better measures are needed for assessing pediatric safety and end-of-life care and few measures are designed for specific age categories among children (Beal et al. 2004).

In the previous section, we considered how medicine's silence on how depression affects men has led to questions about whether men are receiving proper health care. An analogous example in pediatric health care might be the lack of discussion of gender-specific factors that contribute to pediatric conditions. It is interesting to note that the "health topics" found on the American Academy of Pediatrics website are, as Nobelius and Wainer (2004, 11) would say, "gender-blind" and do not include gender-specific topics. For instance, discussion about violence in dating on the website speaks in gender-neutral ways. There are good reasons to hold that violence in dating affects more adolescent girls than adolescent boys because girls are often physically less able to defend themselves (although that certainly is beginning to change). Beyond this, there are numerous gender-specific conditions in pediatric heath care that all call out for attention. As pediatrician George Lazarus says, "[s]exual differentiation in utero affects more than the external and internal sex organs. The brain is a sexual organ and some of the behavioral differences observed between boys and girls (and men and women) are likely due to the effects of androgens on the male brain before birth" (2010, 2). There are good reasons to think that there are gender-specific differences in ADHD, asthma, autism, obesity, and violence that impacts health. Neither are children "miniature adults," nor are boys the same as girls.

Alternatively, with regard to boys, there is a reported underdiagnosis of neurological injuries that occur in sports. Concussions that occur in American football in middle-school and high-school sports have become a significant source of concern (Mayo Clinic 2011). A concussion is a brain injury that can affect memory, speech, and muscle coordination and can cause permanent disability or death. According to Kohn, a "[c]oncussion can be especially serious for children, who are more likely than adults both to sustain a concussion and to take longer to recover. These factors may affect return-to-play decisions, which determine when it is safe for an athlete to participate in sports again" (2010, 1). Despite significant changes in the guidelines that govern middle-school and high-school sports, coaches are usually not able properly to diagnose head injuries, and children and adolescents are reportedly not receiving the medical attention that may help avert future neurological problems. Further, a discussion of gender-specific considerations here may contribute to a reevaluation of our assumptions that "boys will be boys" as they engage in sports that lead to traumas and injuries that are sustained in their lives.

Whereas adolescent girls may be underdiagnosed with clinical problems associated with violence in dating, they may be overdiagnosed with premenstrual syndrome (PMS). As Claman and Miller report, "[p]remenstrual syndrome (PMS), a common cyclic disorder occurring in up to 40% of reproductive-aged women, is characterized by emotional and physical symptoms consistently occurring during the menstrual cycle's luteal phase (the phase that begins with ovulation and ends with the onset of menses).

Studies indicate that 14% to 88% of adolescent girls have moderate-to-severe symptoms of PMS" (Claman and Miller 2006, 329). As we discussed in Chapter 5, a first challenge will be to reevaluate what is meant by PMS in the diagnostic setting. Further, given that up to 88% of adolescent girls are diagnosed with PMS, that hormone therapy is an option for PMS, and that hormone therapy (i.e., birth control) carries significant side effects, an extended discussion about the diagnosis and treatment of PMS in adolescent girls is warranted.

Alternatively, boys may be overdiagnosed with attention deficit hyperactivity disorder (ADHD). Literature reports that ADHD occurs more frequently in boys than girls, with a ratio of three to one (Hermens 2005). Some claim that boys are simply diagnosed more frequently with ADHD than girls in part because girls show fewer aggressive and impulsive symptoms and have lower rates of conduct disorders in school and institutional settings (ADHD in women 2008). Some put it this way, "girls get help while boys get Ritalin." Sixty percent of children diagnosed with ADHD retain the diagnosis as adults (National Institute of Neurological 2008). In 1957, Ritalin (or methylphenidate) became available and prescriptions rose dramatically in early 1990 from 2.5 million to 11 million in 1999, to more than 33 million in 2004 (Miller 2008). Medication sales in the U.S. for ADHD added up to more than 2.7 billion in 2004 and 3 billion in 2006 (Miller 2008), the most popular of which was Ritalin. It is no wonder that some say that Ritalin is the "fourth 'R' in schools." Some ask whether the medical establishment is overprescribing Ritalin to a generation of boys that tend to be active and in need of a different educational system than what is offered by large classrooms in which homogenous conduct is necessary in order to preserve order (Miller 2008).

The cases here illustrate how appropriate gender considerations may fail to operate in pediatric health care. Certainly more can be said, on par with the more extensive development found in the earlier chapters on women's health care. Suffice it to say that pediatric health care has an opportunity to take on important work in gender-specific medicine. Although social class and race/ethnicity have been the primary focus of child health disparities research, evidence is available that a wider range of social, economic, psychosocial, and community factors also contributes to systematic differences in children's health. According to Kandyce Larson et al. (2008), "[r]isk factors including single-parent families, family conflict, maternal mental health and depression, lack of health insurance, and levels of community violence have been shown to predict the prevalence and severity of different child health conditions with some association that is independent from family income, education, or race/ethnicity" (Larson et al. 2008, 337). Such empirical work has led to the development of new conceptual models of children's health that account for the broad range of child, family, and community influences on health and the cumulative toll that multiple co-occurring risk factors may take on children's health. I take Larson et al.

to support gender-specific pediatric medical research on grounds that an integrative approach to pediatric health care is important and gender represents an important "factor" that contributes to the prevalence and severity of different pediatric health conditions.

Gender-specific medicine has an opportunity to develop new models of diagnosis, prognosis, and treatment for conditions that uniquely affect girls and boys (Lazarus 2010). It has the opportunity to challenge assumptions and claims about children and the disease that particularly affect them as it adopts new nomenclature and taxonomies in pediatric health care. As we learned in Chapter 6, the categories of gender and sex already assume a structure of clinical reality and we may not be able to rethink the assumptions and claims that frame them without changing the categories or lenses themselves. Pediatric health care might consider moving beyond the language of "female" and "girl," and "male" and "boy," and use the language of underlying genetic and endocrine factors along with their phenotypical expressions which contribute to the conditions that patients bring to the attention of health care professionals. Rethinking the assumptions and claims made about being "female" or "girl," and "male" or "boy," will influence how medicine thinks about pediatric diseases with a focus on how gender contributes to disease expression and treatment. In the end, reflection upon the character of gender-specific disease has implications in pediatric health care.

IMPLICATIONS FOR MEMBERS OF THE LESBIAN, GAY, BISEXUAL, AND TRANSGENDER COMMUNITIES

Another group that has gone underrepresented in this study comprises members of the lesbian, gay, bisexual, and transgender (LGBT) communities. To begin with, the LGBT populations are anything but uniform. "Like the general United States population, LGBT people are diverse in terms of cultural background, ethnic or racial identity, age, education, income, and place of residence. The degree to which sexual orientation or gender identity is central to one's self-definition, the level of affiliation with other LGBT people, and the rejection or acceptance of societal stereotypes and prejudice vary greatly among individuals" (Gay and Lesbian Medical Association 2000; also see Institute of Medicine 2011). Given such diversity, part of the difficulty in studying the health of members of the LGBT communities is defining what constitutes LGBT individuals. "Lesbian, gay, and bisexual (LGB) people are defined by their sexual orientation, a definition that is complex and variable. Throughout history and among cultures the definition of sexual orientation shifts and changes" (Gay and Lesbian Medical Association 2000). Today, " a generally-accepted definition of lesbian, gay, and bisexual is orientation toward people of the same gender in sexual behavior, affection or attraction, and/or self-identity as gay/lesbian or bisexual" (Gay and Lesbian Medical Association 2000). Definitions and scope of transgender populations are even less adequately researched.

In the previous section, we considered how medicine's silence on how gender-specific factors contribute to pediatric conditions has led to questions about whether children are receiving proper clinical care. An analogous example in LGBT's health care is the lack of discussion and research designed to advance knowledge of LGBT's health. In its report entitled *The Health of Lesbian, Gay, Bisexual, and Transgender People: Building a Foundation for Better Understanding*, the Institute of Medicine (2011) reports that health research of LGBT individuals is woefully lacking. According to the Institute of Medicine, more work is needed on suicide, depression, substance abuse, violence and victimization, the long-term use of hormones for transgender persons, sex reassignment surgeries, the diagnosis of disorders of sex development (DSD), unneeded surgeries for those diagnosed with DSD, and misdiagnoses based on LGBT stereotypes. The most important constraint limiting knowledge concerning the health of lesbian, gay, bisexual, and transgender people is the collection of data from large national on-going population-based surveys funded by the federal government. But even before large-scale research can be done, as previously mentioned, there is a prior challenge to standardize sexual orientation and gender-identity-scale measures employed in such research. As the Institute of Medicine reports, "[e]xisting measures of sexual orientation and gender identity are used differently in various studies depending on the research question" (Institute of Medicine 2011, 7–10). Currently there are "no generally accepted and well-validated set of questions that can cover a variety of situations, including studies among different age cohorts, surveys that focus on topics other than sexual behavior, and research in which participants may not understand terms such as 'gender identity'" (Institute of Medicine 2011, 7–10).

Although there is a need for research and the standardization of gender-identity measures in research on LGBT's health, there is an overemphasis on certain conditions that affect members of the LGBT communities. In particular, a recent survey has found that medical students in the U.S. receive only about five hours of education on LGBT issues (Gay and Lesbian Medical Association 2011). Further, LGBT's health issues are usually raised in the context of sexual and infectious disease discussions, thereby fueling the stereotype that LGBTs are riddled with sexual and infectious diseases. LGBT health issues usually only come up in the clinical curriculum when discussing sexually transmitted diseases or HIV infection and AIDS. Although there are certainly concerns about the vulnerability of certain members of the LGBT community to HIV and AIDS because of the way HIV most effectively enters the bloodstream, it is inaccurate to suggest that *all* members of the LGBT are vulnerable.

Certainly more can be said about how LGBT's health is understood in medicine on par with a more extensive analysis of women's health found in the earlier chapters. But that is a matter for another time. At this point we can say that the health of members of the LGBT communities needs more attention in clinical research and practice. Gender-specific medicine has an opportunity to develop new models of diagnosis, prognosis, and treatment for conditions that uniquely affect members of the LGBT communities. It has the opportunity to challenge assumptions and claims about lesbians, gays, bisexuals, and transgenders and the diseases that particularly affect them as it adopts new nomenclature and taxonomies in LGBT health care. As we learned in Chapter 6, the categories of "female" and "woman," and "male" and "man," already assume a structure of clinical reality and we may not be able to rethink the assumptions and claims that frame them without changing the categories or lenses themselves. LGBT health care might consider moving beyond the language of "lesbian," "gay," "bisexual," and "transgender" and use the language of underlying genotypical and phenotypical factors that contribute to the conditions that patients bring to the attention of health care professionals. Rethinking the assumptions and claims made about being "lesbian," "gay," "bisexual," and "transgender" in medicine will influence how medicine thinks about the health of members of the LGBT communities with a focus on how gender contributes to disease expression and treatment. In the end, reflection upon the character of gender-specific disease has implications in LGBT's health care.

SUMMARY

Gender-specific medicine is not just about women. Its focus on how gender-specific factors contribute to disease expression and treatment has implications for men, children, and members of the LGBT communities. There are good reasons for gender-specific medicine to devote attention to men, girls, boys, lesbians, gays, bisexuals, and transgenders. Such attention is bound to shed further light on how medicine understands gender, disease, and their relation. Building a more solid basis for gender-specific health concerns will add to the repository of health information that pertains to all people. In the end, all patients are bound to benefit from such research because all patients are gendered. But they may not be gendered in ways that we have previously assumed.

10 Some Lessons and Challenges

SUMMING UP

There are a number of lessons that can be drawn from this analysis of the ethics of framing gender-specific disease. These include recognizing that (1) there is need for philosophical investigation of gender-specific disease, (2) gender-specific disease and related bioethical discourses are integrative, (3) an integrative account of gender-specific disease carries implications for how we understand gender, disease, and their relation, and (4) our understanding of gender-specific disease and related bioethical analysis are limited and open to change. In this chapter, each of these lessons will be considered. There are also a number of challenges that can be drawn from this analysis of gender-specific disease. The challenges that are considered include the problem of (1) pluralism, (2) bias, (3) gender imperialism, and (4) gender contagion. In drawing this analysis to a close, it becomes evident that there is more work to be done on the ethics of framing gender-specific disease.

LESSONS LEARNED

A first lesson that one can draw from this inquiry is that there is a need for philosophical investigation of gender-specific disease. As this project illustrates, a philosophical discourse about gender-specific disease is critical to the accuracy of how we understand gender-specific disease. It assists in uncovering, clarifying, and critiquing the claims and assumptions that frame medical concepts and their uses. Such a philosophical approach is part of a long history of analysis in the philosophy of medicine of submitting medical concepts to investigation.

By philosophy of medicine, I mean a philosophical discipline that investigates how we know and act in medicine in order to uncover the claims, assumptions, and practices that frame the discussions (Pellegrino and Thomasma 1981; Wulff 1986; Engelhardt 1977, 1986; Stempsey 2004; Marcum 2008; Johansson and Lynøe 2008). As a philosophical endeavor, it moves beyond set disciplinary boundaries or fields and finds shared interests among foci of study, such as philosophy, medicine, biology, psychology, sociology, and women's studies, thereby creating new perspectives, strategies, and research methodologies that shape and critique knowledge and translate meaning across disciplines. It is a discipline within philosophy defined by "a systematic set of ways for articulating, clarifying, and addressing the philosophical issues in medicine" (Pellegrino and Thomasma 1981, 28). It entails ontological, epistemological, and ethical analyses of our understandings and actions in medicine.

My view that philosophy of medicine is a discipline worthy of pursuit is not held by all. Philosopher Jerome Shaffer (1975, 218) argues that philosophy of medicine is simply the aggregate of studies found in philosophy of science, philosophy of mind, and moral philosophy and that, as a result, "there is nothing left for Philosophy of Medicine to do" (Shaffer 1975, 218). Bioethicist Arthur L. Caplan holds that philosophy of medicine is not a field or discipline because it lacks the breadth, canon, and intellectual challenges typical of a recognized area of study (Caplan, 1992, 72–73). In contrast, my view (Cutter 2003, 8) is that philosophy of medicine offers a unique framework for exploring the ontological, epistemological, and ethical dimensions of medical knowledge and practice. It offers an interdisciplinary approach in order to analyze and assess the nature of medical ideas, how we think we know them, and the practices and goals that inform them. Topics include health and disease, conceptions of the body and mind, models of medicine and clinical judgment, epistemological standards of medical evidence and causation, the health care provider-patient relationship, and related bioethical issues (Pellegrino and Thomasma 1981; Khushf 1997; Schaffner and Engelhardt 1998; Lindemann 1999; Stempsey 2004; Evans et al. 2004; Marcum 2008; Johansson and Lynøe 2008).

Physician-philosophers from Hippocrates (fifth c. B.C.E), Aristotle (384–322 B.C.E), and Galen (approx. 130–210 C.E.) through Edmund D. Pellegrino (1976, 1978) and H. Tristram Engelhardt, Jr. (1977, 1986) have concerned themselves with philosophical analyses of medicine. Hippocrates (1943) is noted for rejecting supernatural explanations about health and disease and emphasizing the role of observation in medical diagnosis, thus associating him with the Aristotelian school of thought, leading him to claims that we still take seriously today. Aristotle (384–322 B.C.E.), the son of a physician, believed that medicine could aid in philosophic and moral tasks to a large degree (Owens 1977). Galen of Pergamum (1968) spent much time developing his theory of humors in order to explain health and disease. English physician Thomas Sydenham (1624–1689) (Romanell 1974, 69–91) advocated for a more rigorous empirical methodology in medicine and encouraged clinicians to classify disease in order to develop better diagnostic and therapeutic guidelines in the clinic. English physician Thomas Percival (1740–1804) (1803) introduced the term "medical ethics" into the vocabulary and insisted that the duties granted to doctors by society are forms of "public trusts." Today, Edmund D. Pellegrino (1976, 1978, 2004), H. Tristram Engelhardt, Jr. (1977, 1981 [1975], 1986), Kenneth

Schaffner (1993), and William Stempsey (2004) are part of an emerging tradition of physicians trained in philosophy who have been instrumental in reenergizing discussions in philosophy of medicine.

The tradition of philosophy of medicine is not simply of historical interest. As Foucault tells us in *Discipline and Punish*, the past is not just the past. It is a "history of the present" (Foucault 1995 [1975], 31) and, I would add, future; it is both memory and forecast, reflections of ourselves, and road maps for future directions of action and change. How we understand medical concepts today is in part a reflection of how we have understood and employed them in the past and present. In that light, philosophy of medicine as a philosophical endeavor lodged in historical discussions allows us to step back and investigate clinical conditions (such as disease and health) and clinical status (such as gendered patients and research subjects) in order to uncover the claims, assumptions, and practices that frame the discussions with an eye toward future developments. Although a philosophical analysis of gender-specific disease certainly does not replace basic and applied scientific work in gender-specific medicine, a philosophical investigation provides a critical role in thinking about, assessing, and guiding such endeavors.

A second lesson is that gender-specific disease and related bioethical discourses are integrative. This is because the *descriptive* role of gender and disease in medicine is inextricably tied to its *prescriptive* role. Descriptions, observations, or the "facts" of gender-specific disease are always ordered around theoretical assumptions, including judgments about how to select and organize evidence into explanations. Further, such descriptions are always ordered around prescriptive or evaluative judgments, including those concerning what objects are assigned significance and what actions are appropriate and warranted in order to achieve certain goals. Clinical descriptions are singled out as worthy of focus and intervention for purposes of achieving numerous and, at times, competing goals. These values or goals in gender-specific medicine include minimizing pain and suffering, returning a patient to biological and/or psychological functioning, meeting patient demands, satisfying professional interests, securing funding, developing health policies, ensuring financial reimbursement, maintaining cultural and social norms, and so on. Still further, gender-specific descriptions and prescriptions are located in particular contexts. There are no timeless or non-contextual accounts of gender-specific disease, or at least there are no such interpretations available to humans.

Yet, given the methodological tools of medicine, the limits of nature, and our shared values, all is not relative. There are still ways we can classify and describe gender-specific disease. Gender-specific disease is integrative in that it defies any attempt to see gender simply as a biological or social phenomenon, disease simply as a biomedical discovery or social construction, and the relation between gender and disease simply as a function of a single causal relation or an open-ended relationship. In contexts in which ethical questions are raised about its use in practice, the notion of gender-specific disease defies any attempt to be analyzed strictly through a bioethical approach that focuses simply on a gender-neutral sense of patient's rights or welfare or on a gender-inclusive sense of choice or welfare that sees gender as a single, static, independent variable. Thus, bioethical discourse about gender-specific disease is integrative.

This brings us to a third lesson. An integrative account of gender-specific disease carries implications for how we understand gender, disease, and their relation. As stated above, gender-specific disease is integrative in that it defies attempts to see gender or disease simply as a biomedical discovery or social construction, and the relation between gender and disease simply as a function of a single causal relation or an open-ended relationship. Gender is neither a simple function of a discoverable biological variable that is detached from its linguistic and cultural contexts, nor is it a simple social construction detached from the physical world. Gender (e.g., "woman," "man," "girl," "boy," "lesbian," "gay," "bisexual, "transgender") is more nuanced, more complex, and more of a continuum than a static dualist social state reflecting one's sex. We can say the same about sex (e.g., "female," "male," and "intersexual"). Sex is more nuanced, more complex, and more of a continuum than a static dualist biological state undergirding one's gender. Further, disease is neither a simple function of discoverable biological function that is detached from its linguistic and cultural contexts, nor is it a simple social construction created by diagnosticians. Disease is a multi-factorial phenomenon brought about by biological dysfunction and interpreted within clinical, psychological, cultural, and social contexts. It functions as a warrant for clinical treatment and is usually seen to be a disvalue. A causal relation between gender and disease is based on various senses of causality, including necessary, sufficient, contributory, and manipulatory. A causal relation between gender and disease is an expression of how gender-specific factors and disease expression are sequentially ordered, how prior events influence those that follow, how certain events can be manipulated in order to bring about other events, and how certain events are valued over others.

Given these conclusions, our current assumptions and claims about gender, disease, and their relation need rethinking. Such rethinking will likely lead to revisions in gender-specific taxonomy and nomenclature. Such will require careful deliberation involving an interdisciplinary team made up of clinical practitioners, researchers, and patients to ensure that the taxonomies and nomenclature are not only epistemologically accurate but clinically useful. Gender-specific medicine will want to use language that reflects proper medical informatics in research and clinical practice, be cautious about asserting that sex-specific diagnoses determine gender-assignments, avoid terms that are misleading or misunderstood, focus on clinical conditions rather than the assumed gender assignment of the person, use language that is clear to both clinicians and patients, and recognize that diagnosis may not dictate therapy (especially as diagnoses are developed and may change as new knowledge is acquired). We can expect that we will be encouraged to move beyond the language of "gender" (e.g., "woman," "man," "girl," "boy," "lesbian," "gay," "bisexual," and "transgender") and "sex" (e.g., "female," "male," and "intersex") and employ alternative language of appropriate genotypical and phenotypical variations that are evident in nature and our interpretations thereof. Still-in-all, new taxonomies and nomenclature will need to be submitted to philosophical analysis in order to tease out problems, especially those concerning deterministic and reductionistic claims. So, caution is advised as new taxonomies and nomenclature are developed to talk about crucial and complex gender-specific notions in medicine.

A fourth lesson is to recognize that our understanding of gender-specific disease and related bioethical discourses are limited and open to change. Let's face it: we all have a tough time accepting uncertainty in medicine. When we go to doctors, we expect infallible experts, we expect immediate diagnoses, and we expect to be cured. But as we so often realize, medicine does not and cannot deliver diagnoses and treatments in this way. As medical attorney and psychiatrist Jay Katz said years ago about medicine in general, "[m]edical knowledge is engulfed and infiltrated with uncertainty. . . . Yet the reality of medical uncertainty is generally brushed aside as doctors move from its theoretical contemplation to its clinical application in therapy and, even more so, in talking with their patients" (Katz 1984, 35). Resistance to acknowledging uncertainty to patients "is also reinforced by the traditional authoritarian relationship that governs interactions between physicians and patients and that doctors seek to foster. Professing certainty serves purposes of maintaining professional power and control over the medical decision-making process as well as of maintaining an aura of infallibility" (Katz 1984, 42). Weeding out suppositions, clarifying what is known and not known, and communicating the uncertainty of gender-specific clinical information should be part and parcel of the task of the gender-specific practitioner when talking about gender-specific disease.

The recognition that our understanding of gender-specific disease is limited and open to change contributes to an invitation to rethink some of the taxonomies and nomenclature in gender-specific medicine. We are reminded of Juengst's suggestions about revisiting the language of clinical diagnostics and Tuana's reminder that what we don't know or do not care to know tells us something about how we think and others think we should think. In the end, there will be situations in which certain taxonomies and language will be preferred over others. Discussion will likely take place, and there will likely be multiple responses offered. If there are willing parties, dialogue will take place and agreement will be sought. If resources permit, dialogue and research will continue and it may be possible to attempt multiple resolutions simultaneously. When resources are scarce, which they typically are, compromise will be the only option short of using force to resolve the conflict. But the compromise itself is bound to be challenged, and when it fails, another one may surface as an alternative. In a sense, every compromise is an invitation to find another one, so there is a process of reconfiguration of options as situations arise, more data become available, and there is evidence that certain options are more beneficial than others. In short, uncertainty is not only part and parcel of human knowing, it is an opportunity to rethink our assumptions and claims.

CHALLENGES POSED

There are a number of challenges posed by this inquiry. These include the problem of (1) pluralism, (2) bias, (3) gender imperialism, and (4) gender contagion. I'll treat each in turn.

First, to what extent does the recognition of pluralism in the ontological, epistemological, and axiological character of gender-specific disease risk relativism and the undermining of useful and reliable gender-specific descriptions and prescriptions? We'll begin with a brief overview of pluralism. Pluralism in epistemology is the position that there is not one consistent set of truths about the world, but rather many. There are different senses of pluralism that can be distinguished. In the case of epistemological pluralism, the position claims that because there is no definitive way to carve up the world into parts, there will be several mutually exclusive complete and true descriptions of the world. In the case of cultural pluralism (see Benedict 1961), the position claims that because truth is relative to a culture, there will be several mutually exclusive complete and true descriptions of the world. In the case of philosophical pragmatism (see James 1981 [1907]), the position claims that because truth is connected to successful action, and success is connected to the goals set by our interests, the correct set of truths will be relative to our interests. Further, pluralism in ethics or morality is the idea that there are several values that may be equally correct and fundamental, and yet they may be in conflict with each other (Beauchamp 1982, 43ff). Moral pluralism postulates that in many cases, such incompatible values may be incommensurable, in the sense that there is no clear objective ordering of them in terms of importance (MacIntyre 1984).

Given this, one might ask to what extent does the recognition of pluralism in our understanding of gender-specific disease undermine the possibility of useful and reliable clinical descriptions and prescriptions? As has already been argued (see Chapter 4), the pluralism that is evident in our understanding of gender-specific disease and related bioethical analyses is to be distinguished from relativism. In gender-specific medicine, we do not completely make up gender-specific disease. In morality, psychological and social phenomena limit the pluralism that characterizes gender-specific medical claims and prevent them from becoming relative. Put positively, a pluralist approach to gender-specific disease and related bioethical discourses does not reduce to a relativist one. It instead highlights the contextually dependent character of the claims made in medicine (see Chapter 4). In this way, a pluralist view of gender-specific disease does not undermine the possibility of useful and reliable gender-specific clinical descriptions and prescriptions.

Second, to what extent do the simultaneous critique and defense of bias or partiality in philosophical discourse on gender matters in medicine risk illogical thinking and the undermining of current practices in medicine? We addressed this concern in an earlier chapter (see Chapter 5) in the context of race- and class-based thinking. We will address this here with regard to gender. The problem of bias or partiality arises from the tension between rejecting partiality and embracing it in order to achieve a certain end. In the case of gender-based thinking, feminist philosopher Louise Antony (2002) puts the problem this way: "On the one hand, it is one of the central aims of feminist scholarship to expose the male-centered assumptions and interests—the male *biases*, in other words—underlying so much of received 'wisdom.' But on the other hand, there is an equally important strain of feminist theory that seeks to challenge the ideal of pure objectivity by emphasizing both the ubiquity and the value of certain kinds of partiality and interestedness" (Antony 2002, 114). Applied here, this study of gender-specific disease has critiqued traditional biased ways of understanding gender, disease, and their relation. At the same time, it has rejected the possibility of achieving a strictly objective, impartial, essentialist view of gender, disease, and their relation in the clinical setting. Given this, can we reject and at the same time support partiality? How is it that *that* bias is problematic but *this* one is permissible?

To address the problem of partiality, I borrow a distinction offered by Elizabeth Anderson (2009), that is, bias as error versus bias as resource. In the foregoing, we have seen numerous examples of how medicine has ignored women and gender issues (e.g., in the early years of AIDS), how research into sex differences and women's and men's "natures" reinforces gender stereotypes and sexist practices in medicine (e.g., in the case of treating menopausal symptoms), and how the applications of medicine and technology disadvantage women in receiving proper care (e.g., in the case of heart disease). In all of these instances, bias has been the cause for *error* in recognizing truth or accuracy in medical claims and, in the case of medical care, what benefits and harms patients.

In contrast, we have seen examples of medical inquiries informed by "legitimate, generative limiting bias" (Anderson 2009). We have seen numerous examples of how medicine has incorporated gender into its framing of disease (e.g., Legato's ground-breaking two-volume set on gender-specific disease), how research into sex and gender differences and women's and men's natures challenges gender stereotypes and sexist practices in medicine (e.g., in the case of hormone therapy), and how the applications of medicine and technology advantage women and other vulnerable groups (e.g., in the case of intersectional studies on smoking-related lung cancer). In these cases, gender bias is the cause for *resourceful* avenues of seeking truth or accuracy. Here what constitutes "resourceful" is key. As Antony says, "[w]hat makes a *good* bias good is that it facilitates the search for truth, and what makes the *bad* bias bad is that it impedes it" (Antony 2002, 115). A major way to assess truth in medicine is through quantitative and qualitative means and the extent to which patient welfare is enhanced and patient harm is minimized. In the case of gender-specific disease, a judgment of good versus bad bias, then, depends on the determination of whether actions result in advancing welfare and minimizing harms to individuals or groups of patients and, if so, to what extent.

Third, to what extent does the recognition that gender matters in disease risk "gender imperialism," the view that because gender is central to understanding disease, all diseases are best conceptualized as gender-specific diseases? Juengst (2004, 244) raises this concern in the context of understanding genetic disease and his point has relevancy in our discussion of gender-specific disease. As this study has shown, given that sex is "in every cell" (Institute of Medicine 2001a, 28), it could easily follow that a project like this encourages us to understand all diseases as sex-based. Given that sex is what we call the biological component of gender, it follows that *all* disease is gender-specific. If all disease is gender-specific, then any account or approach to disease that is not gender-specific is problematic and needs to be revised. Here the problem of gender imperialism arises.

If one understands this project to advise that all clinical classifications ought to be gender-specific, then the charge of gender imperialism is a fair accusation. And I'll admit, the more one takes a gender-inclusive view of disease, the more one is intrigued by differences in health status reported by practitioners and patients. But gender imperialism has not been supported by the earlier analysis. Given the integrative way gender-specific disease has been understood, the project does not support the view that all disease is gender-specific (although medicine can certainly do a much better job in understanding how gender influences disease expression and treatment). There will be some diseases that lend themselves to gender-specific interpretations and treatments, such as X-linked genetic conditions, heart disease, and osteoporosis. Others will be less so, such as broken bones (unless, of course, the bones are those of a woman with advanced osteoporosis). Thus, the call to recognize gender-specific disease is not imperialistic. It is rather a request to investigate whether gender makes a difference in disease expression and treatment, and if so, then to consider ways to develop better diagnostics and treatments in medicine.

Fourth, to what extent does the recognition that gender matters in disease risk "gender contagion," the view that conceptualizing health problems as gender-specific means understanding gender as a specific cause of the problem, leading to the view that "my gender caused my disease" or "my gender made me sick"? Again, I draw from Juengst (2004, 244) in his discussion of genetic disease and apply it to our discussions of gender-specific disease. Gender-specific contagion is the view that conceptualizing disease as gender-specific means understanding gender as a specific cause of the problem, much as the germ theory isolated microbes as the pathogens for infectious disease. It further entails the problem we discussed in an earlier chapter, namely, the problem of determinism, i.e., assuming that gender-specific diagnoses have more predictive power than other kinds of health risk information, as in the case of claiming that "I am destined to be diseased because of my gender."

If one understands this project to advise that all clinical classifications be gender-specific, and that gender is a category that can serve the role akin to an infectious microbe, then indeed it is a fair accusation. But this has not been supported by the earlier analysis. If one understands the project to support a more nuanced view of gender, disease, and their relation, then the accusation of gender contagion is unfounded. Given that the project has explicitly supported a more nuanced view of gender, disease, and their relation, and rejected a reductionist view that gender causes disease, the accusation of gender contagion is unfounded. Gender defies being reduced to a microbe. Gender is an integrative concept involving genotypical and phenotypical factors set within particular frames of reference.

SUMMARY

Our investigation into the ethics of gender-specific disease leads us to appreciate the need for philosophical analysis of gender-specific disease, that gender-specific disease and related bioethical analysis are integrative, that an integrative account of gender-specific disease carries epistemological and ethical implications for how we understand gender, disease, and their relation, and that our understanding of gender-specific disease is limited and open to change. Our investigation also leads us to appreciate the challenges raised in understanding gender-specific disease. These include the problem of pluralism, bias, gender imperialism, and gender contagion. Reflection upon how we think about gender-specific disease will not solve all of the ethical problems in gender-specific health care, but it is a step in the direction of being less vulnerable to committing conceptual errors in understanding gender, disease, and their relation, errors that carry significant ethical implications in the lives of patients.

11 Concluding Reflections

The most common question I have been asked during the writing of this project is: "What difference does gender make in disease expression and treatment?" This chapter addresses this question as it brings the analysis to a close and illustrates why a philosophical consideration of gender-specific disease makes much-needed sense.

Gender makes a difference in disease expression and treatment in four ways. First, it makes a difference biologically. Gender, or rather gender-specific factors, can be shown to lead to differences in how members of particular genders express disease. Disease can vary in terms of signs, symptoms, frequency, progression, and outcome. In order to arrive at evidence to support such differences, clinicians and researchers need to study such phenomena. They need to include members of particular genders in their research studies and carefully map out the variables that define different expressions of disease and its treatment. As we have learned from this study, in such activities clinicians and researchers will want to clarify and define what is meant by gender, disease, and their relation. As this study has shown, this will be no small task. Gender as well as sex is more complex than a static concept that comes in two kinds, disease more complex than simple biological dysfunction, and the relation between gender and disease more complex than a single causal relation. The latter two claims about disease and disease causation will probably not raise much controversy beyond isolated debates; rethinking gender as well as sex will raise significant debate inside and outside the walls of medicine because of our entrenched views about gender and sex, femininity and masculinity, and what constitutes female and male.

Second, gender makes a practical difference in disease expression and treatment. Gender-specific factors can be shown to lead to differences in disease expression and treatment among members of particular genders. When this is recognized, diagnoses, prognoses, and treatment recommendations for particular diseases will change to reflect new knowledge about diseases. In turn, admission forms, clinical texts, clinical coding systems, clinical models, educational curricula, health care delivery systems, and health care policies change as gender-specific medical knowledge and practice becomes more mainstream. The move from a gender-blind to gen-der-inclusive perspective in medicine will be time-consuming and involve significant structural adjustments in health care, how it is funded, and how it is practiced. As medicine changed in light of new knowledge about infectious disease in the beginning of the twentieth century, medicine will change in the beginning of the twenty-first century in light of new knowl-edge in gender-specific medicine.

Third, gender makes an ethical difference in disease expression and treatment. When gender-specific factors can be shown to lead to differ-ences in disease expression and treatment, the ethical mandate in medicine to promote patient autonomy and welfare garners new focus. New knowl-edge in gender-specific medicine comes with new responsibilities to disclose information to patients and revise recommendations for treatment. It comes with new responsibilities to promote patient welfare and minimize patient harm. It comes with new ethical responsibilities to rethink what we mean by patient autonomy and welfare and the bioethical approaches that are commonly used. It comes with new ethical responsibilities to rethink how medicine understands gender, disease, and their relation, and how clinical nomenclature and taxonomies make a difference, sometimes for good and sometimes for bad, in the lives of patients.

This leads us to the fourth way in which gender makes a difference in disease expression and treatment. It makes a difference integratively. That is, in medicine gender can no longer be seen to be an isolated variable in medicine. Gender is inextricably tied to other variables or dimensions of analysis, such as sex, race, ethnicity, socio-economic status, class, and age. There are no sexless genders, and there are no genderless sexes. There are no ethnically neutral, economically neutral, or age-neutral genders. Gender is a dimension of analysis in disease expression and treatment that inte-grates with other dimensions of difference. The challenge will be to design research studies to study this integration at the intersection. The challenge will be to navigate between the boundaries of appropriate and inappropri-ate gender appeals to gender in disease. The challenge will be to convince those footing the bill that gender studies are not just women's studies. Gen-der-specific medicine has the opportunity to work with integrative medi-cine and move medicine into the twenty-first century.

So, yes, Hippocrates (fifth c. B.C.E.) (2005, 62) was correct well before his time: gender matters in disease expression and treatment. As we have learned in this study, it matters biologically, practically, ethically, and inte-gratively. That is, gender matters in disease expression and treatment, in how we structure the health care delivery system and research projects, in how we assess moral responsibility in medicine, and in how we under-stand ourselves as gendered beings. This recognition of the multiplicity and heterogeneity of viewpoints is not new in medicine or bioethics. We already have a medical-industrial complex that supports numerous special-ties and disciplines that take on a wide range of clinical problems, often from differing perspectives. Although the multiplicity and heterogeneity of perspectives may frustrate us (no one likes competing clinical recommendations on a clinical problem), living within and between perspectives is our reality as patients, as health care professionals, and as gendered beings. We already have at our disposal a wide range of interpretations of gender, disease, disease causation, and bioethical methodologies that support numerous perspectives on a host of clinical issues. Such is not simply an academic exercise, but a thoroughly human one of judging, evaluating, and hoping for something better in our lives in the different ways in which we do so. It is one that recognizes the limitations of our knowledge and the ways in which we seek to overcome such limitations through discourse and a rethinking of our cherished views.

In the end, we accept that gender-specific medical theories and practices are only approximations to the truth, and their trustworthiness depends on the extent to which they have been exposed to critical experiments. The more they are exposed, the more they can be trusted. We are left with a sense of the problems that we have inherited and problems that we may wish to avoid. The challenge is to resist retreating from the problems because of fear that "the solution is too complex," "the solution won't work," "there's no money," "they won't be convinced," or "that's too controversial." Small steps can make a difference—and small steps accessed critically are needed in order to advance our thinking about gender-specific disease in the twenty-first century. They are needed in order to advance gender-specific medical practice, an endeavor that carries significant implications in the lives of women, men, girls, boys, lesbians, gays, bisexuals, and transgenders, or whatever our terminology will be—in other words, all of us.

Bibliography

Achterberg, Jeanne. 1991. *Woman as healer: A panoramic survey of the healing activities of women from prehistoric times to the present.* Boston, Massachusetts: Shambhala.

Acocella, Joan. 1998. The politics of hysteria. *The New Yorker* April 6: 64–79.

ADHD in women. 2008. *Medscape today.* www.medscape.com/viewarticle/515209 (accessed February 29, 2008).

Agich, George. 1997. Toward a pragmatic theory of disease. In *What is disease?,* edited by J.M. Humber and R.F. Almeder, 221–46. New Jersey: Humana Press.

Alcoff, Linda. 2006. *Visible identities.* New York: Oxford University Press.

American Academy of Pediatrics. 2011. AAP fact sheet. http://www.aap.org/visit/facts.htm (accessed June 8, 2011).

American College of Physicians/American Society of Internal Medicine. 2001. Reasons for sex-specific and gender-specific study of health topics. *Annals of internal medicine* 135 (10): 935–38.

American Psychiatric Association. 1952. *Diagnostic and statistical manual of behavioral disorders.* Washington, D.C.: American Psychiatric Association.

American Psychiatric Association. 1968. *Diagnostic and statistical manual of behavioral disorders.* 2nd ed. Washington, D.C.: American Psychiatric Association.

American Psychiatric Association. 1980. *Diagnostic and statistical manual of behavioral disorders.* 3rd ed. Washington, D.C.: American Psychiatric Association.

American Psychiatric Association. 1987. *Diagnostic and statistical manual of behavioral disorders.* 3rd ed. rev. Washington, D.C.: American Psychiatric Association.

American Psychiatric Association. 1994. *Diagnostic and statistical manual of behavioral disorders.* 4th ed. Washington, D.C.: American Psychiatric Association.

American Psychiatric Association. 2000. *Diagnostic and statistical manual of behavioral disorders.* 4th ed. rev. Washington, D.C.: American Psychiatric Association.

American Society of Plastic Surgeons Overall Trends. 2008. http://www.plasticocsurgery.org/medicine/statistics/loader.cfm?url=/commonspot/securit/getfile.cfm+PageID=29287 (accessed May 4, 2009).

Anderson, Elizabeth. 2009. Feminist epistemology and philosophy of science. *Stanford encyclopedia of philosophy.* http://plato.stanford.edu/entries/feminism-epistemology (accessed December 1, 2009).

Annis, David. 1978. A contextual theory of epistemic justification. *American philosophical quarterly* 15: 213–19.

Antony, L.M. 2002. Quine as feminist: The radical import of naturalized episte-mology. In *A mind of one's own*, edited by L.M. Antony and C.E. Witt, 110–53. Boulder, Colorado: Westview Press.

Aristotle. 1941. *Nicomachean ethics*. In *The basic works of Aristotle*, translated by W.D. Ross, and edited with an introduction by R. McKeon, 927–1112. New York: Random House.

Aristotle. 1984. *On the generation of animals*. In *The complete works of Aristotle*, translated by A. Platt, edited by J. Barne, Vol. 8, 665–83. New Jersey: Princeton University Press.

Arizona Center for Integrative Medicine. 2009. What is IM? http://integrative-medicine.arizona.edu/about/index.html (accessed December 15, 2009).

Astin, John A. and Kelly Forys. 2004. Psychosocial determinants of health and illness: Reintegrating mind, body, and spirit. In *Integrative medicine: Princi-ples for practice*, edited by B. Kligler and R. Lee, 25–36. New York: McGraw-Hill.

Auto Workers v. Johnson Controls, Inc. 1991. 499 U.S. 187.

Baier, Annette. 1992. Alternative offerings to Asclepius. *Medical humanities review* 6 (1): 9–19.

Bartlett, Katherine T. 1990. Feminist legal methods. In *Feminist legal theory*, edited by D.K. Weisberg, 383–93. Pennsylvania: Temple University Press.

Bassuk, Shari S. and JoAnn E. Manson. 2004. Gender and its impact on risk fac-tors for cardiovascular disease. In *Principles of gender-specific medicine*, edited by M.J. Legato, 193–214. Amsterdam/Boston: Elsevier.

Beal, Anne C. et al. 2004. Quality measures for children's health care. *Pediatrics* 113 (Supp 1): 199–209.

Beauchamp, Tom L. 1982. *Philosophical ethics: An introduction to moral philoso-phy*. New York: McGraw Hill Book Co.

Beauchamp, Tom L. and James F. Childress. 2009 (1979). *Principles of biomedical ethics*. 6th ed. New York: Oxford University Press.

Beeghley, Leonard. 2004. *The structure of social stratification in the United States*. New York: Pearson.

Bender, Frederic L. 2003. *The culture of extinction*. New York: Prometheus.

Benedict, Ruth. 1961. Relativism and patterns of culture. In *Value and obligation*, edited by R.B. Brandt, 450–99. New York: Harcourt, Brace, and World.

Bentham, Jeremy. 1996. *An introduction to the principles of morals and legisla-tion*, edited by J.H. Burns and H.L.A. Hart. Oxford: Clarendon.

Berenson, Alex. 2005. Sale of impotence drugs fall, defining expectations. *The New York Times*. http://74.125.155.132/scholar?q=cache:cBZcXtALDXoJ:sc holar.google.com/+sales+of+viagra++Berenson&hl=en&as_sdt=0,6 (accessed April 4, 2011).

Bertranpetit, Jaume and Francesc Calafell. 2007. Genetic and geographical vari-ability in cystic fibrosis: Evolutionary considerations. In *Ciba Foundation symposium: Variation in the human genome*, edited by D. Chadwick and G. Cardew. http://www3.interscience.wiley.com/cgi-bin/summary (accessed Janu-ary 23, 2008).

Bethell, Christina D. et al. 2011. A national and state profile of leading health problems and health care quality for US children: Key insurance disparities and across-state variations. *Academic Pediatrics* 11 (3) (Supp 1): S22–S33.

Bichat, Xavier. 1981 (1801). Pathological anatomy: Preliminary discourse. In *Concepts of health and disease: Interdisciplinary perspectives*, edited by A.L. Caplan et al., 167–73. Massachusetts: Addison-Wesley Publishing Company.

Bickel, Janet. 2000. *Women in medicine: Getting in, growing, and advancing*. California: Sage Publications.

Bird, Chloe E. and Patricia P. Rieker. 2008. *Gender and health: The effects of constrained choices and social policies.* Massachusetts: Cambridge University Press.
Blumenthal, Susan J. and Jessica Kagan. 2002. The effects of socioeconomic status on health in rural and urban America. *Journal of the American medical association* 287 (1): 109.
Bono, Chaz. 2011. *Transition: The story of how I became a man.* New York: Dutton Adult.
Boorse, Christopher. 1975. On the distinction between health and disease. *Philosophy and public affairs* 5: 49–68.
Boorse, Christopher. 1977. Health as a theoretical concept. *Philosophy of science* 44: 542–73.
Boorse, Christopher. 1997. A rebuttal on health. In *What is disease?*, edited by J.M. Humber and R.F. Almeder, 3–171. New York: Humana Press.
Bordo, Susan. 1990. Feminism, postmodernism, and gender skepticism. In *Feminism/postmodernism*, edited by L.J. Nicholson, 152. New York: Routledge.
Boston Women's Health Book Collective. 1973. *Our bodies, ourselves.* New York: Simon and Schuster.
Boston Women's Health Collective. 1998. *Our bodies, ourselves for the new century.* 3rd ed. New York: Simon and Schuster.
Bowman, Inci. 1976. Classification of diseases: Part 1. *The bookman* 3 (6): 1–10.
Brody, Howard. 1994. My story is broken: Can you help me fix it? Medicine ethics and the joint construction of narrative. *Literature and medicine* 13: 79–92.
Broussais, F.J.V. 1981 (1828). *Examen des doctrines medicales et des systems de nosologie.* Paris: Megvignon-Marvis.
Broverman, I.K. et al. 1970. Sex-role stereotypes and clinical judgements of mental health. *Journal of consulting and clinical psychology* 34: 1–7.
Bullough, V. and M. Voght. 1973. Women, menstruation, and 19th century medicine. *Bulletin of the history of medicine* XLVII: 67–80.
Butler, Judith. 1990. *Gender trouble.* New York: Routledge.
Butler, Judith. 1993. *Bodies that matter.* New York: Routledge.
Byrne, William. 2004. Central nervous system. In *Principles of gender-specific medicine*, edited by M.J. Legato, 61. Amsterdam/Boston: Elsevier.
Canguilhelm, Georges. 1978 (1966). *On the normal and the pathological*, translated by C.R. Fawcett. Holland: D. Reidel Publishing Company.
Caplan, Arthur L. 1992. Does the philosophy of medicine exist? *Theoretical medicine* 13: 67–77.
Caplan, Arthur L. et al., eds. 1981. *Concepts of health and disease: Interdisciplinary perspectives.* Massachusetts: Addison-Wesley Publishing Company.
Caplan, Arthur L. et al., eds. 2004. *Health, disease, and illness: Concepts in medicine.* Washington, D.C.: Georgetown University Press.
Cartwright, Samuel A. 1981 (1851). Report on the diseases and physical peculiarities of the negro race. In *Concepts of health and disease: Interdisciplinary perspectives*, edited by A.L. Caplan et al., 305–32. Massachusetts: Addison-Wesley Publishing Company.
Centers for Disease Control. 1981a. Kaposi sarcoma and pneumocystic pneumonia among homosexual men—New York City and California. *Morbidity and mortality weekly report* 30: 305–8.
Centers for Disease Control. 1981b. Pneumoncystic pneumonia—Los Angeles. *Morbidity and mortality weekly report* 30: 250–52.
Centers for Disease Control. 1982. Update on acquired immune deficiency syndrome (AIDS)—United States. *Morbidity and mortality report* 31: 507–14.
Centers for Disease Control. 1992. 1993 revised classification system for HIV infection and expanded surveillance case definition for AIDS among adolescents and adults. *Morbidity and mortality weekly report* 41: 1–19.

Centers for Disease Control and Prevention. 2006. Leading cases of death: Males—United States, 2002. www.cdc.gov/men/Icod.htm (accessed June 6, 2007).

Centers for Disease Control and Prevention. 2011. Injury prevention and control: Violence prevention. http://www.cdc.gov/ViolencePrevention/index.html (accessed May 15, 2011).

Chodorow, Nancy. 1978. *The reproduction of mothering: Psychoanalysis and the sociology of gender.* Berkeley: University of California Press.

Claman, Faith and Terri Miller. 2006. Premenstrual syndrome and premenstrual dysphoric disorder in adolescence. *Journal of pediatric health care* 20 (5): 329–33.

Cleveland Clinic. 2008. Depression in men. *The Cleveland Clinic Health Information Center.* www.clevelandclinic.org/health/health-info/docs (accessed February 21, 2008).

Cohen, Stewart. 1999. Contextualism, skepticism, and the structure of reasons. *Philosophical Perspectives* 13: 57–89.

Collingwood, R. 1940. *An essay on metaphysics.* Oxford: Clarendon Press.

Collins, Karen Scott et al. 1999. *Health concerns across a woman's lifespan. The Commonwealth Fund 1998 survey of women's health.* New York: Commonwealth Fund.

Color blindness. 2011. *Medline plus.* www.nlm.nih.gov/medlineplus/colorblindness.html.

Conrad, Peter. 2007. *The medicalization of society: On the transformation of human conditions into treatable disorders.* Maryland: Johns Hopkins University Press.

Corea, Gena. 1992. *The invisible epidemic: The story of women and AIDS.* New York: Harper Collins.

Cornell, Drucilla. 2004. Gender in America. In *Keywords: Gender—for a different kind of globalization*, edited by N. Tazi, 33–54. New York: Other Press.

Council on Ethical and Judicial Affairs, American Medical Association. 1991. Gender disparities in clinical decision making. *Journal of the American medical association* 266, 560–64.

Council on Graduate Medical Education, U.S. Department of Health and Human Services. 1996. *Fifth report: Women and medicine.* Rockville, Maryland: Council on Graduate Medical Education.

Cowley, G. and K. Springen. 2002. The end of the age of estrogen? *Newsweek* July 22: 38–41.

Crenshaw, Kimberlé Williams. 1991. Mapping the margins: Intersectionality, identity politics, and violence again women of color. *Stanford law review* 43: 1241–99.

Culture specific diseases. 2007. http://anthro.palomar.edu/medical/med_4htm (accessed April 15 2008).

Cutter, Mary Ann Gardell. 1989. Explaining AIDS: A case study. In *The meaning of aids: Perspectives from the humanities*, edited by E. T. Juengst and B. Koenig, 21–29. New York: Praeger Scientific.

Cutter, Mary Ann Gardell. 1990. Negotiating criteria and setting limits: The case of AIDS. *Theoretical Medicine* 11 (September): 193–200.

Cutter, Mary Ann Gardell. 1992. Value presuppositions in diagnosis: A case study of cervical cancer. In *The ethics of diagnosis*, edited by J.L. Peset et al., 147–54. Holland: Kluwer Academic Publishers.

Cutter, Mary Ann Gardell. 1997. Engelhardt's analysis of disease: Implications for a feminist epistemology. In *Reading Engelhardt*, edited by B. Minogue, 139–48. Holland: Kluwer Academic Publishers.

Cutter, Mary Ann Gardell. 2003. *Reframing disease contextually.* Holland: Kluwer Academic Publishers.

Cutter, Mary Ann Gardell 2006. On women's health care: In search of nature and norms. In *The death of metaphysics; The death of culture*, edited by M. Cherry, 199–217. Holland: Springer Academic Publishers.

Daniels, Jessie and Amy J. Schulz. 2006. Constructing whiteness in health disparities research. In *Gender, race, class, and health: Intersectional approaches*, edited by A.J. Schultz and L. Mullings, 89–127. California: Jossey-Bass.

de Beauvoir, Simone. 1952. *The second sex*, translated and edited by H.M. Parshley. New York: Alfred A. Knopf.

DeLorey, Catherine. 2007. Health care reform—A woman's issue. *National women's health network* December 31. *www.nwhn.org/wha_marapr07_healthcarereform* (accessed December 31, 2007).

Department of Gender, Women, and Health, World Health Organization. 2007. www.who.int/gender/en/index.html (accessed June 18, 2007).

Department of Health and Human Services. 1985. *Women's health: Report of the public health service task force on women's issues*. Vols. 1 and 2. Washington, D.C.: Public Health Service.

Department of Health and Human Services. 2006. Summary health statistics for U.S. adults: National health interview survey, 2004. Washington, D.C.: Department of Health and Human Services.

Department of Health and Human Services. 2011. *National health expenditure data*. http://www.cms.hhs.gov/NationalHealthExpendData/25_NHE_Fact_Sheet.asp#TopOfPage (accessed July 31, 2011).

DeRose, Keith. 1992. Contextualism and knowledge attributions. *Philosophy and Phenomenological research* 52 (4): 913–29.

Diamond, Jed. 2004. *The irritable male syndrome: Managing the four key causes of depression and aggression*. Pennsylvania: Rodale Books.

Donchin, Anne. 2009. Feminist ethics. *Stanford encyclopedia of philosophy*. http://plato.stanford.edu/entries/feministbioethics (accessed August 1, 2009).

Dreger, Alice Domurat. 1998. *Hermaphrodites and the medical invention of sex*. Massachusetts: Harvard University Press.

Dreger, Alice Domurat. 2004. Ambiguous sex—or ambivalent medicine? In *Health, disease, and illness: Concepts in medicine*, edited by A.L. Caplan et al., 137–52. Washington, D.C.: Georgetown University Press.

Dreger, Alice D. et al. 2005. Changing the nomenclature/taxonomy for intersex: A scientific and clinical rationale. *Journal of pediatric endocrinology and metabolism* 18: 729–33.

Dresser, Rebecca. 1992. Wanted: Single, white male for medical research. *Hastings center report* Jan/Feb: 24–29.

Dresser, Rebecca. 1996. What bioethics can learn from the women's health movement. In *Feminism and bioethics: Beyond reproduction*, edited by S.M. Wolf, 144–59. New York: Oxford University Press.

Duesberg, Peter. 1994. Infectious AIDS—Stretching the germ theory beyond its limits. *International archives of allergy and immunology* 103 (2): 118–27.

Eisenberg, D.M. et al. 1998. Trends in alternative medicine use in the United States, 1990–1997: Results of a follow-up national survey. *Journal of the American medical association* 280 (18): 1569–75.

Engel, George L. 1981 (1977). The need for a new medical model: A challenge for biomedicine. In *Concepts of health and disease: Interdisciplinary perspectives*, edited by A.L. Caplan et al., 589–607. Massachusetts: Addison-Wesley Publishing Company.

Engelhardt, H. Tristram, Jr. 1977. Is there a philosophy of medicine? *PSA 1976* 2: 94–108.

Engelhardt, H. Tristram, Jr. 1981 (1975). The concepts of health and disease. In *Concepts of health and disease: Interdisciplinary perspectives*, edited by A.L. Caplan et al., 31–46. Massachusetts: Addison-Wesley Publishing Company.

Engelhardt, H. Tristram, Jr. 1982 . The subordination of the clinic. In *Value conflicts in health care delivery*, edited by B. Gruzolski and C. Nelson, 41–57. Massachusetts: Ballinger.

Engelhardt, H. Tristram, Jr. 1986. From philosophy *and* medicine to philosophy *of* medicine. *Journal of medicine and philosophy* 11: 3–8.

Engelhardt, H. Tristram, Jr. 1996. *Foundations of bioethics*. 2nd ed. New York: Oxford University Press.

Engelhardt, H. Tristram, Jr. and Kevin W. Wildes. 2003. Health and disease: Philosophical perspectives. *Encyclopedia of bioethics*, edited by S.G. Post, 1101–6. 3rd ed. New York: Macmillian Reference Books.

Evans, Martyn et al. 2004. *Philosophy for medicine: Applications in a clinical context*. Oxford: Radcliffe Medical Press.

Faber, K. 1923. *Nosology in modern internal medicine*. London: Humphrey Milford.

Faden, Ruth et al. 1996. Women as vessels and vectors: Lessons from the HIV epidemic. In *Feminism and bioethics: Beyond reproduction,* edited by S. Wolf, 266–78. New York: Oxford University Press.

Farmer, Paul. E. et al. 2006. Structural violence and clinical medicine. *PLoS Med* 3 (10): e449. doi:10.1371/journal.pmed.0030449. http://www.plosmedicine.org/article/info%3Adoi%2F10.1371%2Fjournal.pmed.0030449

Fauci, Anthony. 1993. Multifactorial nature of immunodeficiency syndrome virus disease: Implications for therapy. *Science* 3136: 1011–18.

Fausto-Sterling, Anne. 1993. The five sexes: Why males and female are not enough. *The sciences* March/April: 20–24.

Fausto-Sterling, Anne. 2000a. The five sexes revisited. *The sciences* July/August: 18–23.

Fausto-Sterling, Anne. 2000b. *Sexing the body: Gender politics and the construction of sexuality*. New York: Basic Books.

Fausto-Sterling, Anne. 2005 The bare bones of sex: Part 1—Sex and gender. *Signs* 30: 1491–1527.

Federation of Feminist Women's Health Centers. 1981. *A new view of a women's body*. New York: Simon and Schuster.

Flanagin, Annette and Margaret A. Winkler. 2006. Theme issue on poverty and human development. *Journal of the American medical association* 296 (24). www.jama.ama-assn.org/cgi/content/full/296/24/2970 (accessed January 15, 2006).

Fleck, Ludwik. 1979 (1935). *Genesis and development of a scientific fact,* translated by F. Bradley and T.J. Trenn, edited by T.J. Trenn and R.K. Merton. Chicago: University of Chicago Press.

Food and Drug Administration. 1992. FDA clinical testing guidelines will represent women. *Food drug letter* 20: 424.

Food and Drug Administration. 1993. *Guidelines for the study and evaluation of gender differences in the clinical evaluation of drugs*. Washington, D.C.: Food and Drug Administration.

Foot, Philippa. 1958–59. Moral beliefs. *Proceedings of the Aristotelian society* 59, 83–104.

Foucault, Michel. 1973 (1963). *Birth of the clinic: An archeology of medical perception,* translated by A.M. Sheridan Smith. New York: Pantheon Books.

Foucault, Michel. 1978. *The history of sexuality: An introduction,* translated by Robert Hurley. New York: Pantheon.

Foucault, Michel. 1995 (1975). *Discipline and punish: The birth of the prison,* translated by Alan Sheridan. New York: Vintage Books.

Friedman, Marilyn. 2003. *Autonomy, gender, and politics*. New York: Oxford UniversityPress.

Fugh-Berman, Adriane. 2005. Why race-based medicine is a bad idea. *National women's health network* September/October. *www.nwhn.org/wha_septoct05_rxchange* (accessed December 31, 2007).

Galen. 1968. *On the usefulness of the parts of the body*, translated by M.T. May. New York: Cornell University Press.

Gallo, Robert C. and Luc Montagnier. 1987. The chronology of AIDS research. *Nature* 326 (6112): 435–36.

Garcia-Moreno, Claudia et al. 2006. Prevalence of intimate partner violence: Findings from the WHO multi-country study on women's health and domestic violence. *The lancet* 368 (9543): 1260–69, October 7. doi:10.1016/S0140–6736(06)69523–8 . *http://www.thelancet.com/journals/lancet/article/PIIS0140–6736(06)69523–8/fulltext* (accessed May 1, 2011).

Garrison, H. 1929. *An introduction to the history of medicine*. 4th ed. Philadelphia: Saunders.

Gay and Lesbian Medical Association and Columbia University Joseph L. Mailman School of Public Health Center for Lesbian, Gay, Bisexual, and Transgender Health. 2000. Lesbian, gay, bisexual, and transgender health: Findings and concerns. http://www.dialog.unimelb.edu.au/project/links/pdf/glma%20white%20paper%20jan%2000.pdf (accessed May 23, 2011).

Gay and Lesbian Medical Association. 2011. http://glma.org (accessed August 22, 2011).

Gender medicine. 2011. Multimedia healthcare. www.mmhc.com (accessed August 4, 2008).

Gilbert, Dennis. 1998. *The American class structure*. New York: Wadsworth Publishing Company.

Gilligan, Carol, 1982. *In a different voice*. Massachusetts: Harvard University Press.

Girman, Andrea et al. 2004. Integrative approaches to common conditions in women's health. In *Integrative medicine: Principles for practice*, edited by B. Kligler and R. Lee, 763–87. New York: McGraw-Hill.

Glezerman, Marek. 2010. Forward. In *Principles of gender-specific medicine*, edited by M.J. Legato, xvii–xx. Amsterdam/Boston: Elsevier.

Goldsmith, Marsha F. 1992. Specific HIV-related problems of women gain more attention at a price affecting more women. *Journal of the American medical association* 268: 1814–16.

Goosens, William K. 1980. Values, health, and medicine. *Philosophy of science* 47: 100–15.

Gøtzsche, Peter C. 2007. *Rational diagnosis and treatment: Evidence-based clinical decision-making*. 4th ed. England: John Wiley and Sons, Ltd.

Gould, Stephen Jay. 1981. *The mismeasure of man*. New York: Norton.

Greenspan, Miriam. 1993. *A new approach to women and therapy*. Pennsylvania: TAB Books.

Griswold v. Connecticut. 1965. 381 U.S. 479.

Hacking, Ian. 1999. *Social construction of what?* Massachusetts: Harvard University Press.

Harding, Sandra. 1986. *The science question in feminism*. New York: Cornell University Press.

Harding, Sandra. 1991. *Whose science? Whose knowledge?* New York: Cornell University Press.

Hare, R.M. 1952. *The language of morals*. England: Oxford University Press.

Hartsock, Nancy. 1983. *Money, sex, and power: Toward a feminist historical materialism*. Boston: Longman.

Hartsock, Nancy. 1998. *The feminist standpoint revisited and other essays.* Colorado: Westview Press, 1998.

Haugen, Aage. 2002. Women who smoke: Are women more susceptible to tobacco-induced lung cancer? *Carcinogenesis* 23 (2): 227–29.

Hegel, G.W.F. 1970 (1830). *Philosophy of nature,* translated by M.J. Petry. London: Allen and Urwin.

Henrich, Janet B. and Catherine M. Viscoli. 2006. What do medical schools teach about women's health and gender differences? *Academic medicine* 81 (5): 476–82.

Hermens, D.F. 2005. Sex differences in adolescent ADHD: Findings from concurrent EEG and EDA. *Clinical Neurophysiology* 116 (6): 1455–63.

Heron, Melonie. 2010. Deaths: Leading causes for 2006. *National Vital Statistics Reports* 58, (14), March 31. http://www.cdc.gov/nchs/data/nvsr/nvsr58/nvsr58_14.pdf (accessed January 4, 2011).

Hersh, A.L. et al. 2004. National use of postmenopausal hormone therapy. *Journal of the American medical association* 291: 47–53.

Hickey, Joseph and William Thompson. 2007. *Society in focus.* California: Allyn and Bacon.

Hippocrates. 1923. *Hippocrates,* Vol. 1, translated by W.H. Jones. Massachusetts: Harvard University Press.

Hippocrates. 1943. *Regimen,* translated by W.H.S. Jones. Massachusetts: Harvard University Press.

Hippocrates. 2005. *The Hippocratic corpus.* In *Women's life in Greece and Rome,* 3rd ed., edited by M. Lefkowitz and M. Fant, 230–43. Maryland: Johns Hopkins University Press.

Hirschbein, Laura D. 2006. Science, gender, and the emergence of depression in American Psychiatry. *Journal of the history of medicine and allied sciences* 61 (2): 187–216.

Hoagland, Sarah Lucia. 1989. *Lesbian ethics.* California: Institute of Lesbian Studies.

Holmes, H.B. and L.M. Purdy, eds. 1992. *Feminist perspectives in medical ethics.* Indiana: Indiana University Press.

Houck, Judith A. 2006. *Hot and bothered: Women, medicine, and menopause in modern America.* Cambridge, Massachusetts: Harvard University Press.

Hubbard, Ruth. 2004. Rethinking woman's biology. In *Race, class, and gender in the United States,* 6th ed., edited by P.S. Rothenberg, 65–68. New York: Worth Publishers.

Hughes, Ieuan A. et al. 2006. Consensus statement on management of intersex disorders. *Archives of disease in childhood* 91: 554–62.

Humber, J.M. and R.F. Almeder, eds. 1997. *What is disease?* New York: Humana Press.

Hume, David. 1978 (1739–40). *Treatise of human nature,* edited by L.A. Selby-Brigge and revised by P.H. Nidditch. England: Oxford University Press.

Hyde, Janet Shipley and Beverly Whipple. 2005. Synthesis: Overarching themes and future directions for research. In *Biological substrates of human sexuality,* edited by J.S. Hyde, 171–78. Washington, D.C.: American Psychological Association.

Institute of Medicine. 2001a. *Exploring the biological contributions to human health: Does sex matter?,* edited by T. Wizemann and M. Pardue. Washington, D.C.: National Academy Press.

Institute of Medicine. 2001b. *Health and behavior: The interplay of biological, behavioral, and social influences.* Washington, D.C.: National Academy Press.

Institute of Medicine. 2011. *The health of lesbian, gay, bisexual, and transgender people: Building a foundation for better understanding.* Washington D.C.: National Academies Press.

International Association of Feminist Approaches to Bioethics. 2011. www.fabnet.org (accessed January 15, 2011).

Intersex Society of North America. 2011 (2008). How common is intersex? http://www.isna.org/faq/frequency (accessed January 6, 2011).

Jackson, Pamela Braby and David R. Williams. 2006. The intersection of race, gender, and SES health paradoxes. In *Gender, race, class, and health: Intersectional approaches*, edited by A.J. Schulz and L. Mullings, 131–61. California: Jossey-Bass.

Jaggar, Alison. 1992. Feminist ethics. In *Encyclopedia of ethics*, edited by L. Becker with C. Becker, 363–64. New York: Garland.

James, William. 1981 (1907). *Pragmatism: A new name for some old ways of thinking*. Indiana: Hackett Publishing Company.

Johansson, Ingvar and Niels Lynøe. 2008. *Medicine and philosophy: A twenty-first century introduction*. Frankfurt: Ontos Verlag.

Jonsen, Albert R. 1998. *The birth of bioethics*. New York: Oxford University Press.

Journal of gender-specific medicine. 2008. Published by Elsevier. http://gender-medjournal.com/ (accessed November 8, 2010).

Juengst, Eric. 1995. The ethics of prediction: Genetic risk and the physician-patient relationship. *Genome science and technology* 1 (1): 21–36.

Juengst, Eric. 2004. Concepts of disease after the Human Genome Project. In *Health, disease, and illness: Concepts in medicine*, edited by A.L. Caplan et al., 243–62. Washington, D.C.: Georgetown University Press.

Kant, Immanuel. 1964 (1781/1787). *Critique of pure reason*. New York: St. Martin's Press.

Kant, Immanuel. 1985 (1785). *Foundations of the metaphysics of morals*, translated by L.W. Beck. New York: Macmillan.

Katz, Jay. 1984. Why doctors don't disclose uncertainty. *The Hastings Center report* 10: 35–44.

Kaufman, Frederik. 1997. Disease: Definition and objectivity. In *What is disease?*, edited by J.M. Humber and R.F. Almeder, 269–86. New Jersey: Humana Press.

Kendell, Robert. 1971. The concept of disease. *British journal of psychiatry* 128: 508–9.

Khushf, George. 1997. Why bioethics needs the philosophy of medicine: Some implications of reflection on concepts of health and disease. *Theoretical medicine and bioethics* 18: 145–63.

Khushf, George. 1999. The aesthetics of clinical judgments: Exploring the link between diagnostic elegance and effective resource utilization. *Medicine, health care, and philosophy* 2: 141–59.

King, Lester. 1954. What is disease? *Philosophy of science* 12: 193–203.

King, Lester. 1963. *Growth of medical thought*. Chicago: University of Chicago Press.

King, Lester. 1984. *Medical thinking*. New Jersey: Princeton University Press.

King, Patricia. 1992. The dangers of difference. *The Hastings Center report* 22 (6): 35–38.

Kingsland, Sharon E. 2007. *Maintaining continuity through a scientific revolution: A rereading of E.B. Wilson and T.H. Morgan on sex determination and Mendelism*. Chicago: University of Chicago Press.

Klatt, E.C. 1998. HIV Infection, diagnosis, and treatment: New findings and approaches. *Medical laboratory observer* February: 22–29.

Klausner, Kim. 2005. Intersexuals: Exploding the binary sex system. In *Women's health*, 3rd ed., edited by N. Worcester and M. Whatley, 159–62. Iowa: Kendell/Hunt.

Kligler, Benjamin and Roberta Lee. 2004. *Integrative medicine: Principles for practice.* New York: McGraw-Hill.

Kohlberg, Lawrence. 1984. *Essays on moral development: Vol. 2, the psychology of moral development.* California: Harper and Row.

Kohn, Linda. 2010. *Concussion in high school sports.* Washington, D.C.: U.S. Government Accountability Office.

Koopsen, Cyndie and Caroline Young. 2009. *Integrative health: A holistic approach for health professionals.* Massachusetts: Jones and Bartlett Publishers.

Kramer, Peter. 2005. *Against depression.* New York: Penguin Group.

Kraupl-Taylor, F. 1979. *The concepts of illness, disease, and morbus.* Cambridge: Cambridge University Press.

Kuhn, Thomas S. 1996 (1962). *The structure of scientific revolutions.* Chicago: University of Chicago Press.

Lancaster, T. et al. 2002. Individual counseling for smoking cessation. *Cochrane database of systemic reviews* 3: CD001292.

Landesman, S. and S. Holman. 1995. Epidemiology and natural history of HIV infection in women. In *Primary care of women and children with HIV infection*, edited by P. Kelly et al., 19–35. Boston: Janes and Bartlett Publishers.

Langley, Ricky L. 2004. *Sex and gender differences in health and disease.* North Carolina: Carolina Academic Press.

Laqueur, Thomas. 1990. *Making sex: Body and gender from the Greeks to Freud.* Massachusetts: Harvard University Press.

Larson, Kandyce et al. 2008. Influence of multiple social risks on children's health. *Pediatrics* 121 (2): 337–44.

Lazarus, George M. 2004. Introduction: Gender and development. In *Principles of gender-specific medicine,* edited by M.J. Legato, 1–3. Amsterdam/Boston: Elsevier.

Lazarus, George M. 2010. Introduction: Gender and normal development. In *Principles of gender-specific medicine.* 2nd ed., edited by M.J. Legato, 2. Amsterdam/Boston: Elsevier.

Lee, Roberta et al. 2004. Integrative medicine: Basic principles. In *Integrative medicine: Principles for practice*, edited by B. Kligler and R. Lee, 3–23. New York: McGraw-Hill.

Legato, Marianne J. 2004a. Cardiology. In *Principles of gender-specific medicine,* edited by M.J. Legato, 183–84. Amsterdam/Boston: Elsevier.

Legato, Marianne J. 2004b. Preface. In *Principles of gender-specific medicine,* edited by M.J. Legato, xv–xvi. Amsterdam/Boston: Elsevier.

Legato, Marianne J., ed. 2004c. *Principles of gender-specific medicine.* Vols. 1 and 2. Amsterdam/Boston: Elsevier.

Legato, Marianne J. 2010a. Preface. In *Principles of gender-specific medicine,* edited by M.J. Legato, xxi–xxii. Amsterdam/Boston: Elvesier.

Legato, Marianne J., ed. 2010b. *Principles of gender-specific medicine.* 2nd ed. Amsterdam/Boston: Elvesier.

Legato, Marianne J. and Jaswinder K. Legha. 2004. Gender and the heart: Sex-specific differences in normal myocardial anatomy and physiology and in the experiences of some diseases of the cardiovascular system. In *Principles of gender-specific medicine*, edited by M.J. Legato, 185–92. Amsterdam/Boston: Elsevier.

Lindemann, James. 1999. *Meaning and medicine: A reader in philosophy of health care.* New York: Routledge.

Locke, John. 1980 (1690). *Second treatise of government.* Indiana: Hackett Publishing Company.

Longino, Helen E. 1997. Feminist epistemology as a local epistemology. *The Aristotelian society: Supplementary volume* 71 (1): 19–36.

Lorber, Judith. 1995. Social construction of gender. In *Race, class, and gender in the United States*, 3rd ed., edited by P.S. Rothenberg, 34–36. New York: Worth Publishers.

Lorber, Judith and Lisa Jean Moore. 2002. *Gender and the social construction of illness*. 2nd ed. New York: Rowman Altamira.

MacIntyre, Alastair. 1984. *After virtue*. Indiana: Notre Dame Press.

Mackenzie, Catriona and Natalie Stoljar, eds. 2000. *Relational autonomy: Feminist perspectives on autonomy, agency, and the social self*. New York: Oxford University Press.

Magnus, David. 2004. The concept of genetic disease. In *Health, disease, and illness: Concepts in medicine*, edited by A.L. Caplan et al., 233–42. Washington, D.C.: Georgetown University Press.

Mahowald, Mary. 1993. *Women and children in health care*. New York: Oxford.

Manning, Rita. 1992. *Speaking from the heart*. New York: Rowan and Littlefield.

Marcum, James A. 2008. *An introductory philosophy of medicine: Humanizing modern medicine*. Holland: Springer.

Margolis, Joseph. 1976. The concept of disease. *Journal of medicine and philosophy* 1: 238–55.

Mayo Clinic. 2008. Erectile dysfunction. *Men's health*. www.mayoclinic.com/health/erectile-dysfunction (accessed February 15, 2008).

Mayo Clinic. 2011. Concussion Symptoms. Retrieved from *http://www.mayoclinic.com* (accessed July 15, 2011).

McCrea, Frances B. 2004. The politics of menopause. In *Health, disease, and illness: Concepts in medicine*, edited by A.L. Caplan et al., 187–200. Washington, D.C.: Georgetown University Press.

Merton, Vanessa. 1996. Ethical obstacles to the participation of women in biomedical research. In *Feminism and bioethics: Beyond reproduction*, edited by S.M. Wolf, 216–51. New York: Oxford University Press.

Mikkola, Mari. 2008. Feminist perspectives in sex and gender. *Stanford encyclopedia of philosophy*. http://plato.standford.edu/entries/feminism-gender/ (accessed August 1, 2008).

Mill, John Stuart. 1979 (1861). *Utilitarianism*, edited with an introduction by G. Sher. Indiana: Hackett Publishing Co.

Miller, Toby. 2008. Ritalin: Panic in the USA. *Cultural studies review* 14 (2): 103–12.

Miller, Virginia. 2005. Review of *Principles of gender-specific medicine*. *The Physiologist* 48 (2), April. www.the-aps.org/publications/+p[hys/2005html/AprTPhys/bookreview (accessed October 31 2008).

Moi, Toril. 2001. *What is a woman: Sex, gender, and the body in feminist theory*. Oxford: Oxford University Press.

Moncher, Karen L. and Pamela S. Douglas. 2004. Importance of and barriers to including women in clinical trials. In *Principles of gender-specific medicine*, edited by M.J. Legato, 275–82. Amsterdam/Boston: Elsevier.

Moreno, Jonathan. 1995. *Deciding together: Bioethics and moral consensus* New York: Oxford.

Moreno, Jonathan. 2003. Bioethics is a naturalism. In *Pragmatic Bioethics*, 2nd ed., edited by G. McGee, 3–16. Massachusetts: The MIT Press.

Mullings, Leith and Amy J. Schulz. 2006. Intersectionality and health: An introduction. In *Gender, race, class, and health: Intersectional approaches*, edited by A.L. Schulz and L. Mullings, 3–17. California: Jossey-Bass.

Murphy, Dominic. 2008. Concepts of disease and health. *Stanford encyclopedia of philosophy*. http://plato.stanford.edu/entries/health-disease/ (accessed September 24, 2008).

Murphy, Edmond. 1976. *The logic of medicine*. Maryland: Johns Hopkins University Press.

National Center for Complementary and Alternative Medicine, National Institutes of Health. 2009. Health Info. http://nccam.nih.gov (accessed January 15, 2009).

National Center for Health Care Statistics. 2008a. Health expenditures. www.cdc.gov/nchs/fastats/hexpense.htm (accessed January 23, 2008).

National Center for Health Care Statistics. 2008b. Men's health. www.cdc.goc/nchs/fastats/mens_health.htm (accessed January 29, 2008).

National Center for Health Care Statistics. 2008c. Women's health. *www.cdc.gov/nchs/fastats/womens_health.htm* (accessed January 23, 2008).

National Fragile X Foundation. 2011. What is fragile X? National fragile X foundation. www.fragilex.org (accessed November 4, 2011).

National Institute of Allergy and Infectious Diseases. 1995. *The relationship between the human immunodeficiency virus and the acquired immmunodeficiency syndrome*. Maryland: National Institutes of Health.

National Institute of Mental Health. 2008. Depression in men. www.nimh.nih.gov/health/topics/depression/men_and_depression (accessed February 1, 2008).

National Institute of Neurological Disorders and Stroke. 2008. Attention deficit-hyperactivity disorder information page. www.hihds.hih.gov/adhd (accessed February 28, 2008).

National Kidney and Urologic Disease Information Clearinghouse. 2008. About erectile dysfunction. www.kidney.niddk.nih.gov (accessed February 23, 2008).

National Women's Health Network. 2007. Hypothyroidism: A women's health issue. January/February. *www.nwhn.org/wha_janfeb07_hypothyroidism* (accessed January 25, 2008).

National Women's Health Network. 2009. *The women's health activist*. www.nwhn.org (July 23, 2009).

Nelson, Lynn Hankinson. 2001. *Damaged identities, Narrative repair*. New York: Cornell University Press.

Niranjana, Seemanthini. 2004. Gender in India. In *Keywords: Gender—for a different kind of globalization*, edited by N. Tazi, 133–65. New York: Other Press.

Nobelius, Anne Maree and Jo Wainer. 2004. *Gender and medicine: A conceptual guide for medical educators*. Australia: Monash University School of Rural Health.

Noddings, Nel. 1984. *Caring*. California: University of California Press.

Northrup, Christiane. 2002. *Women's bodies, women's wisdom*. New York: Bantam Books.

Nozick, Robert. 1974. *Anarchy, state, and utopia*. Massachusetts: Harvard University Press.

Oaks, L. 2001. *Smoking and pregnancy: The politics of fetal protection*. New Jersey: Rutgers University Press.

Office of Women's Health, U.S. Department of Health and Human Services. 2007. About us. http://www.4women.gov/OWH/about (accessed June 18, 2007).

Ossorio, Pilar. 2004. Societal and ethical issues in pharmacogenomics. In *Pharmacogenomics: Applications to patient care*, edited by W.L. Allen et al., 399–438. Missouri: American College of Clinical Pharmacology.

Owens, Joseph. 1977. Aristotelian ethics, medicine, and the changing nature of man. In *Philosophical medical ethics: Its nature and significance*, edited by S.F. Spicker and H.T. Engelhardt, Jr., 127–42. Holland: D. Reidel Publishing Company.

Pamuk, Elsie R. et al. 1998. Socioeconomic status and health chartbook. In *Health, United States, 1998*. Maryland: National Center for Health Statistics.

Partnership for Gender-Specific Medicine. 2008. http://partnership.hs.columbia. edu/publications.html (accessed December 8, 2008).

Partnership for Women's Health at Columbia University. 2007. *http://cpmcnet.columbia.edu/dept/partnership/* (accessed November 15, 2007).

Pellegrino, Edmund D. 1976. Philosophy of medicine: Problematic and potential. *The Journal of medicine and philosophy* 1, 5–31.

Pellegrino, Edmund D. 1978. Philosophy of medicine: Towards a definition. *Journal of medicine and philosophy* 11, 9–16.

Pellegrino, Edmund D. 2004. "Forward: Renewing medicine's basic concept" In *Health, disease, and illness: Concepts in medicine,* edited by A.L. Caplan et al., xi–xiv. Washington, D.C.: Georgetown University Press.

Pellegrino, Edmund D. and David C. Thomasma. 1981. *A philosophical basis of medical practice.* New York: Oxford University Press.

Pellegrino, Edmund D. and David C. Thomasma 1988. *For the patient's good: The restoration of beneficence in health care.* New York: Oxford University Press.

Percival, Thomas. 1803. *Medical ethics: Or, a code of institutes and precepts, adapted to the professional conduct of physicians and surgeons.* London: S. Russell.

Perry, Ralph Barton. 1954. *Realm of values: A critique of civilization.* Massachusetts: Harvard University Press.

Pfizer. 2008. About erectile dysfunction. *www.pfizer.com/products/viagra* (accessed February 14, 2008).

Pojman, Louis P. 2003. *The theory of knowledge.* California: Wadsworth/Thomson Learning.

Popper, Karl. 1974. *Conjectures and refutations.* 5th ed. London: Routledge and Kegan Paul.

Porche, Demetrius J. 2007. A call for American journal of men's health. *American journal of men's health* 1 (1): 1–3.

Porche, Demetrius J. and D.G. Willis. 2004. Nursing and men's health movement: Considerations for the 21st century. *Nursing clinics of North America* 39 (2): 251–58.

Potter, Van Rensselaer. 1970. Bioethics: The science of survival. *Perspectives in biology and medicine* 14: 127–53.

Potter, Van Rensselaer. 1971. *Bioethics: Bridge to the future.* New Jersey: Prentice-Hall.

"Pregnant man" gives birth to second child. 2009. *MSNBS* June 11. http://today. msnbc.msn.com/id/31237998 (accessed June 11, 2009).

Price, H.H. 1953. *Thinking and experience.* London: Hutchinson's University Library.

Production of ICD-11: The Revision Process. 2007. http://www.who.int/classifications/icd/ICDRevision.pdf (accessed October 4, 2010).

Purdy, Laura. 1996. A feminist view of health. In *Feminism and bioethics: Beyond reproduction,* edited by S. Wolf, 163–83. New York: Oxford University Press.

Rakel, D. and Andrew Weil. 2007. *Philosophy of integrative medicine.* 2nd ed. Pennsylvania: Saunders Elsevier.

Ratcliff, Kathryn Stother. 2002. *Women and health: Power, technology, inequality, and conflict in a gendered world.* Boston: Allyn and Bacon.

Rawlinson, Mary. 2001. The concept of a feminist bioethics. *Journal of medicine and philosophy* 26 (4): 405–6.

Rawls, John. 1971. *A theory of justice.* Massachusetts: Cambridge University Press.

Reis, Elizabeth. 2007. Divergence or disorder? The politics of naming intersex. *Perspectives in biology and medicine* 50 (4): 535–43.

Results. 2011. Medicaid. *Results: The power to end poverty.* http://www.results. org/issues (accessed August 7, 2011).

Reznek, Lawrie. 1987. *The nature of disease*. London: Routledge and Kegan Paul.
Roberts, Barbara. 2004. Gender-specific aspects of the experience of coronary artery disease. In *Principles of gender-specific medicine*, edited by M.J. Legato, 215–23. Amsterdam/Boston: Elsevier.
Roe v. Wade. 1973. 410 U.S. 113.
Romanell, Patric. 1974. *John Locke and medicine*. New York: Pometheus.
Rosen, Michael R. and Thai Pham. 2004. Impact of gender on the response to cardioactive drugs. In *Principles of gender-specific medicine*, edited by M.J. Legato, 241–54. Amsterdam/Boston: Elsevier.
Ruse, Michael. 2005. Methodological naturalism under attack. *South African journal of philosophy* 24 (1): 44–60.
Ruzek, Sheryl Burt. 1978. *The women's health movement: Feminist alternatives to medical control*. New York: Praeger.
Ruzek, Sheryl Burt and Julie Becker. 1998. The women's health movement in the United States: From grass roots activism to professional agendas. *The journal of the American medical women's association* January 30.
Sassower, Raphael and Mary Ann G. Cutter. 2007. *Ethical choices in contemporary medicine*. England: Acumen.
Sax, Leonard. 2002. How common is intersex?: A response to Anne Fausto-Sterling. *Journal of sex research* 39: 174–79.
Sax, Leonard. 2005. *Why gender matters*. New York: Doubleday.
Schaffner, Kenneth F. 1993. *Discovery and explanation in biology and medicine*. Chicago: University of Chicago Press.
Schaffner, Kenneth F. and H. Tristram Engelhardt, Jr. 1998. Medicine, philosophy of. In *Routledge encyclopedia of philosophy*, Vol. 6, edited by E. Craig, 264–69. New York: Routledge.
Schulz, Amy L. and Leith Mullings, eds. 2006. *Gender, race, class, and health: Intersectional approaches*. California: Jossey-Bass.
Seaman, Barbara. 2003. *The greatest experiment ever performed on women: Exploding the estrogen myth*. New York: Hyperion.
Seldin, Donald. 1977. The medical model: Biomedical sciences as the basis for medicine. In *Beyond Tomorrow*. New York: Rockefeller University Press.
Shaffer, Jerome. 1975. Round-table discussion. In *Evaluation and explanation in the biomedical sciences*, edited by H.T. Engelhardt, Jr. and S.F. Spicker, 215–29. Netherlands: D. Reidel Publishing Company.
Shah, N. 2001. *Contagious divides: Epidemics and race in San Francisco's Chinatown*. California: University of California Press.
Sherwin, Susan. 1992. *No longer patient: Feminist ethics and health care*. Pennsylvania: Temple University Press.
Sherwin, Susan. 2008. Whither bioethics? How feminism can help reorient bioethics. *International journal of feminist approaches to bioethics* 1 (1): 7–27.
Sherwin, Susan et al., eds. 1998. *The politics of women's health: Exploring agency and autonomy*. Philadelphia: Temple University Press.
Shilts, Randy. 1987. *And the band played on: Politics, people, and the AIDS Epidemic*. New York: St. Martin's Press.
Singer, Peter. 1995. *Animal liberation*. 2nd ed. London: Pimlico.
Smith, Donald C. et al. 1975. Association of exogenous estrogen and endometrial carcinoma. *New England journal of medicine* 293: 1164–67.
Smith-Rosenberg, Carroll and Charles Rosenberg. 1981. The female animal: Medical and biological views of woman and her role in nineteenth-century America. In *Concepts of health and disease: An interdisciplinary perspective*, edited by A.L. Caplan et al., 281–303. Massachusetts: Addison-Wesley Publishing Company.
Sommerhoff, G. 1950. *Analytical biology*. London: Oxford University Press.
Sontag, Susan. 1978. *Illness as metaphor*. New York: Farrer, Straus, and Giroux.

Sontag, Susan. 1989. *AIDS and its metaphors.* New York: Farrar, Straus, and Giroux.

Spake, Amanda. 2002. The menopause marketplace. *U.S. news and world report* November 18: 42–50.

Spector, Rachel E. 1996. *Cultural diversity in health and illness.* 4th ed. Connecticut: Appleton and Lange.

Stein, Rachel and Michael Silverstein. 2010. Potential implications of US healthcare reform for American children. In *Archives of disease in childhood.* 2010;archdischild161000 Published online first: April 6, 2010 (accessed July 6, 2011).

Stempsey, William E. 2004. The philosophy of medicine: Development of a discipline. *Medicine, health care, and philosophy* 7: 243–51.

Stoljar, Natalie. 1995. Essence, identity, and the concept of woman. *Philosophical topics* 23: 261–93.

Sundström, Per. 1998. Interpreting the notion that technology is value-neutral. *Medicine, health care, and technology* 1 (1): 41–45.

Sydenham, Thomas. 1981 (1676). Preface to the third edition. In *Concepts of health and Disease: Interdisciplinary perspectives,* edited by A.L. Caplan et al., 145–55. Massachusetts: Addison-Wesley Publishing Company.

Szasz, Thomas. 1961. *Myth of mental illness.* New York: Harper-Hoeber.

Szasz, Thomas. 1991 (1970). *Ideology and insanity.* New York: Syracuse University Press.

Tavris, Carol. 1992. *Mismeasure of woman.* New York: Simon and Schuster.

Tazi, Nadia, ed. 2004. *Keywords: Gender—for a different kind of globalization.* New York: Other Press.

ten Have, Henk and Helen Keasberry. 1992. Equity and solidarity: The context of health care in the Netherlands. *Journal of medicine and philosophy* 17 (August): 463–77.

Thagard, Paul. 1999. *How scientists explain disease.* New Jersey: Princeton University Press.

Tobin, Jonathan N. et al. 1987. Sex bias in considering coronary bypass surgery. *Annuls of internal medicine* 107 (1): 19–25.

Tong, Rosemarie. 1997. *Feminist approaches to bioethics: Theoretical reflections and practical applications.* Colorado: Westview Press.

Tong, Rosemarie. 2004. Feminist perspectives, global bioethics, and the need for moral language translation skills. In *Linking visions,* edited by R. Tong, A. Donchin, and S. Dodds, 89–104. Maryland: Rowman and Littlefield Publishers.

Tong, Rosemarie. 2007. *New perspectives in healthcare ethics: An interdisciplinary and crosscultural approach.* New Jersey: Pearson/Prentice Hall.

Tonneson, Diana. 2006. Reflections: 10 years of courage. *Pause* Fall/Winter: 8–10.

Treichler, Paula A. 1999. *How to have theory in an epidemic: Cultural chronicles of AIDS.* North Carolina: Duke University Press.

Tuana, Nancy. 1988. The weaker seed: The sexist bias of reproductive theory. *Hypatia* 3 (1): 35–59.

Tuana, Nancy. 2006. The spectrum of ignorance: The women's health movement and epistemologies of ignorance. *Hypatia* 21 (3): 1–19.

U.S. Census Bureau. 2008. Race data. *Racial and ethnic classifications used in census 2000 and beyond. http://www.census.gov/populations/socdemo/race/racefactscb.html* (accessed December 16, 2009).

U.S. Census Bureau. 2011. 2011 statistical abstract. *http://www.census.gov/compendia/statab/overview.html* (accessed June 8, 2011).

U.S. Congress Public Law 103–43. 1993. *National institutes of health revitalization amendment.* Washington, D.C.: U.S. Government Printing Office.

United Nations, Office of the High Commissioner for Human Rights. 2004. The right of everyone to the enjoyment of the highest attainable standard of physical and mental health. *United Nations Commission on Human Rights Resolution.* New York: United Nations.

United Nations. 2008a. Concepts and definitions. *Women's watch. www.un.org/ womenwatch/osagi/conceptsanddefinitions.htm* (accessed February 15, 2008).

United Nations. 2008b. Gender mainstreaming. *Women's watch. www.un.org/ womenwatch/osagi/gendermaistreaming.htm* (accessed February 15, 2008).

United Nations Development Programme, Human Development Report. 2006. *Beyond scarcity: Power, poverty, and global water crisis.* http://hdr.undp.org/ hdr2006 (accessed December 7, 2006).

van Hooft, Stan. 1997. Disease and subjectivity. In *What is disease?*, edited by J.M. Humber and R.F. Almeder, 289–323. New York: Humana Press.

Varmus, Harold. 1989. Naming the AIDS virus. In *The meaning of aids: Perspectives from the humanities*, edited by E.T. Juengst and B. Koenig, 3–11. New York: Praeger Scientific.

Virchow, Rudolf. 1981 (1858). One hundred years of general pathology. In *Concepts of health and disease*, edited by A.L. Caplan et al., 190–95. Massachusetts: Addison-Wesley Publishing Company.

Von Wright, G. 1971. *Explanation and understanding.* New York: Cornell University Press.

Waisberg, J. and P. Paige. 1988. Gender role nonconformity and perception of mental illness. *Women's health* 14: 3–16.

Walker, Margaret Urban. 1994. Global feminism: What's the question? *APA newsletter on feminism and philosophy* 94 (1): 53–54.

Walker, Margaret Urban. 1998. *Moral understandings: A feminist study in ethics.* New York: Routledge, 1998.

Walker, Margaret Urban. 2003. *Moral contexts.* Lanham, Maryland: Rowman and Littlefield.

Warner, Jennifer. 2011. Genetic link to lupus. *Web MD.* lupus.webmd.com/ news/20091019 (accessed October 19, 2009).

Wartofsky, Marx. 1976. The mind's eye and the hand's brain: Toward an historical epistemology of medicine. In *Science, ethics, and medicine*, edited by H.T. Engelhardt, Jr. and D. Callahan, 167–94. New York: The Hastings Center.

Weber, Lynn. 2006. Reconstructing the landscape of health disparities research: Promoting dialogue and collaboration between feminist intersectional and biomedical paradigms. In *Gender, race, class, and health: Intersectional approaches*, edited by A.L. Schulz and L. Mullings, 21–59. California: Jossey-Bass.

Weil, Andrew. 1995. *Natural health, natural medicine.* Boston: Houghton Mifflin.

Weil, Andrew. 2004. *Health and healing: The philosophy of integrative medicine and optimum health.* New York: Mariner Books.

Weisfeldt, M. 2004. Preface. In *Principles of gender-specific medicine*, edited by M.J. Legato, xii–xiii. Amsterdam/Boston: Elsevier.

Weissman, Myrna M. and Mark Olfson. 1995. Depression in women: Implications for health care research. *Science* 269: 799–801.

Williams, Michael. 1991. *Unnatural doubts: Epistemological realism and the basis of skepticism.* Massachusetts: Blackwell.

Wilson, Robert A. 1962. The roles of estrogen and progesterone in breast and genital cancer. *Journal of the American medical association* 182: 327–33.

Wilson, Robert A. 1966. *Feminine forever.* New York: M. Evans and Company.

Wittgenstein, Ludwig. 1963. *Philosophical investigations*, translated by G.E.M. Anscombe. Oxford: Basil Blackwell, sec 371.

Wolf, Susan M. 1996. *Feminism and bioethics: Beyond reproduction.* New York: Oxford University Press.

Women's Health Initiative, National Heart, Lung, and Blood Institute. 2007. WHI background and overview. *Women's health initiative.* http://www.nhlbi.nih.gov/whi/background.htm (accessed June 18, 2007).

Woodhouse, Mark B. 1997. The concept of disease in alternative medicine. In *What is disease?*, edited by J.M. Humber and R.F. Almeder, 325–55. New Jersey: Humana Press, Inc.

Worcester, Nancy and Marianne H. Whatley, eds. 2005. *Women's health.* 3rd ed. Iowa: Kendell/Hunt.

World Health Organization. 1958. Constitution. In *The first ten years of the world health organization*, edited by the World Health Organization. Geneva: World Health Organization.

World Health Organization. 1992. *International statistical classification of disease and related health problems*, tenth revision. Geneva: World Health Organization.

World Health Organization. 2007. Poverty and health. *www.who.in/hdp/poverty/en/* (accessed January 20, 2008).

World Health Organization. 2010. What do we mean by 'sex' and 'gender'. http://www.who.int/gender/whatisgender/en/index.html (accessed January 15, 2010).

Worldwide HIV and AIDS Statistic Summary. 2007. www.avert.org/worldstats.htm (accessed January 22, 2008).

Wulff, Henrik R. 1981. *Rational diagnosis and treatment: An introduction to clinical decision-making.* 2nd ed. Oxford: Blackwell Scientific Publications.

Wulff, Henrik R. 1986. *Philosophy of medicine: An introduction.* Oxford: Blackwell Scientific Publications.

Wysowski, D.K. et al. 1995. Use of menopausal estrogens and medroxyprogesterone in the United States 1982–1992. *Obstetrics and gynecology* 85: 6–10.

Young, Iris Marion. 2005. *On female body experience.* New York: Oxford University Press.

Index

For Product Safety Concerns and Information please contact our EU
representative GPSR@taylorandfrancis.com
Taylor & Francis Verlag GmbH, Kaufingerstraße 24, 80331 München, Germany

www.ingramcontent.com/pod-product-compliance
Ingram Content Group UK Ltd.
Pitfield, Milton Keynes, MK11 3LW, UK
UKHW021112180425
457613UK00005B/60

* 9 7 8 0 4 1 5 5 0 9 9 7 8 *